D0881092

Sex, Contraception,
and Motherhood in Jamaica

This volume is published as part of a long-standing cooperative program between Harvard University Press and the Commonwealth Fund, a philanthropic foundation, to encourage the publication of significant and scholarly books in medicine and health.

Sex, Contraception, and Motherhood in Jamaica

Eugene B. Brody

 A COMMONWEALTH FUND BOOK

HARVARD UNIVERSITY PRESS

Cambridge, Massachusetts, and London, England   *1981*

Library of Congress Cataloging in Publication Data

Brody, Eugene B.
    Sex, contraception, and motherhood in Jamaica.

    "A Commonwealth Fund book."
    Bibliography: p.
    Includes index.
    1. Sex customs—Jamaica.   2. Birth control—Jamaica.
3. Adolescent mothers—Jamaica.   4. Unmarried mothers—
Jamaica.   5. Child abuse—Jamaica.   I. Title.
HQ18.J25B76   363.9'6'097292   81-4133
ISBN 0-674-80277-2   AACR2

Acknowledgments

I owe Professor Michael Beaubrun a permanent debt of gratitude for his invitation to come to Jamaica, initially for the period February 1-April 1, 1972, and for his later professional and personal support during my work in his department. Dr. Robert Collis, the World Health Organization psychiatrist assigned to the Jamaican government to whom I was officially responsible, was helpful without fail. My first step in exploring the population issue was to talk with Dr. Wynante Patterson, Principal Government Medical Officer of the National Family Planning Board, the government agency supporting the contraceptive campaign. Dr. Patterson's continued interest was necessary for later developments. Dr. Lenworth Jacobs, founder and President of the Jamaica Family Planning Association (JFPA), also provided much appreciated support and permission to discuss my project with local clinic directors. The most active and easily accessible clinic was that operated by the JFPA at 65 East Street in downtown Kingston, in the center of the old town, Kingston Parish. There I was fortunate to encounter two sympathetic, interested, and actively helpful colleagues, Dr. Carl Stratman, public information officer of JFPA, and Nurse E. Wallace, the senior clinician on daily duty in the clinic. They made it possible for me to conduct the interviews that were basic to formulating a research proposal, approved by the National Family Planning Board and submitted to the Smithsonian Institution for funding. Grateful acknowledgment is made to the Interdisciplinary Communications Project of the Smithsonian for its support. The funds paid for travel, clerical support in Baltimore, and most important, contributed three part-time salaries to Jamaican interviewers. Two recruited by Professor Beaubrun became close and valued colleagues who conducted detailed interviews with our female respondents. Drs. Janet LaGranade and Frank Ottey were at that time registrars in Professor Beaubrun's department. Mr. Ken Byfield, a senior and experienced Health Visitor for JFPA, was selected by Dr. Stratman and staff with the approval of Dr. Jacobs to conduct a series of briefer interviews with male JFPA clients.

Beyond my actual work at the University of the West Indies (UWI) and in the family planning clinics the explorations of other parts of the setting were made possible and enriched immensely by native and adopted Jamaicans who offered me their friendship and knowledge of the island's history, politics, song and story. Among these Dr. Fred Hickling; Brian and Anne Hudson; Anne Garside, an experienced school visitor in Jamaica; and Olive Lewin, founder and director of the National Folksingers of Jamaica, deserve special thanks.

Acknowledgments are also due to Dr. Keith Smith of the University of Maryland's Department of Social and Preventive Medicine, who was a primary statistical consultant for the research, and to the Center for Advanced Study in the Behavioral Sciences, Stanford, California, where with the aid of a grant from the Commonwealth Fund I assimilated my Jamaican experience and analyzed the statistical data. I owe special thanks to Dr. Carol Trainer, the Center's resident statistician, and to Mrs. Agnes Page, my secretary. Upon my return to the University of Maryland, Mrs. Eileen Potocki, my long-time senior secretary, supervised the tasks of manuscript preparation. Without her—as usual—little could have been accomplished.

Contents

1   The Problem   1

2   An Approach to the Problem:
    Epistemological Aspects of Interviewing
    and Clinical Practice in the Field   15

3   The Folk Context of Sex and Reproduction   40

4   The Place:
    Kingston, Metropolis of a Rural Island   62

5   Women without Power: The Social and
    Economic Context of Sex and Reproduction   82

6   Relationship with Mother, Menarche,
    and First Intercourse   120

7   The First Sexual Partnership, the First Pregnancy,
    and the First Child   146

8   Sexual Partnerships, Marriage,
    and Reproductive Behavior   186

9   The Person in the Context   209

10 Public Policy and Private Behavior   231

    References   263

    Index   273

Sex, Contraception,
and Motherhood in Jamaica

1   The Problem

The Human Reproductive Crisis

Reproduction is essential to the survival of any species. It is the fundamental basis for recruiting new members to human society. But like other biological processes necessary to replacement, repair, and diversification—of individuals or populations—it can proliferate to the point of endangering what it evolved to protect. It has already created changes in the density, distribution, and age of the world's population, which in turn have profoundly affected our social and physical environments. These changes threaten the fragile biosphere and—through their influence on developmental experience and family life—the very character of human nature.

Although United Nations data (1980) suggest that the birthrate in developing countries is declining and the desire for large families diminishing, they also indicate that global growth continues. It will not stop (even assuming a continuing and progressive decline in birthrate) until the world's population has nearly tripled from its 1980 level of approximately four billion. The population of the developing world in particular is not expected to stabilize— even with optimal conditions—until near the end of the twenty-first century.

The rapid and extreme human population changes of the nineteenth and twentieth centuries stem mainly from technology. Public health and medical technology have reduced miscarriages, infant mortality, and the infectious diseases of childhood and adolescence so that—in the absence of abortion—conception is more apt than ever before to result in a human being who will become a reproductively capable adult. The technology of food production and distribution contributes to earlier sexual maturity. Earlier menarche and the appearance of secondary sex characteristics mean earlier sexual intercourse, pregnancy, childbirth, and a longer reproductive career. It is true that famine, regarded by some as a corrective imposed by population density upon fertility, does reduce birthrates. Moderate, chronic malnutrition, however, has only a minimal negative effect on fertility, less important than the poverty-linked social or behavioral factors that stimulate it (Bongaarts, 1980). India, for example, with one-seventh of the world's population, contains approximately half the world's chronically undernourished people. They are too poor to afford even the minimum diet necessary to sustain moderate activity levels (Brookings, 1980, p. 14). It is clear that the quality of life for these people is not the same as for those who have adequate food. Yet the Indian population continues to increase at an annual rate of about 2.2 percent. This growth is supported by agricultural technology, which results in an annual increase in food grain production of approximately 2.8 percent, comparable with that of the developed world (Sanderson and Roy, 1979).

The technologies of transportation and communication have also contributed to the human reproductive crisis by stimulating aspirations that cannot be achieved in mainly rural home settings. To the old migratory push of drought, hunger, poverty, boredom, and lack of opportunity for self and children has been added the pull of urban areas, with their promise not only of panaceas for these problems but also of excitement and freedom (Brody, 1970, 1973). Transportation has made global migration from resource-poor to richer areas possible on an unprecedented scale.

Some migration, international as well as internal, is circular; individuals seek work and live in temporary quarters pending their return home, even though that return may not be expected for years. The reproductive consequences of their sexuality, in social and developmental terms, are uncertain. Much migration, though, especially from countryside to city within the same nation, involves entire families or young people intending to establish new permanent homes or to create new families.

War and political oppression also contribute to the problems of displacement and resettlement. The world's roadways and seaways are filled with refugees, for whom the difficulties of reestablishing themselves as productive members of a new community are sometimes almost insurmountable. As the birthrates of long-industrialized countries decline, their populations are increased by those from less developed nations in which reproductive performance and birthrates remain high.

In the still developing world, in particular, settlements have mushroomed around major urban centers. These centers continue to grow in a disorderly way inimical to the quality of human experience. United Nations forecasts predict that by the year 2000 there will be 61 cities with populations of more than 4 million people each. In Latin America, where the great cities are already rimmed with squatters' colonies containing more people than the official urban areas themselves, there are projections of 31 million for Mexico City and 26 million for Sao Paulo; in Asia, Shanghai is expected to have 24 million and Peking 21 million inhabitants.

What are some of the consequences of extreme and rapid human population growth and the migration corollary to it?

Famine is one potential consequence, although in absolute terms it may be no more serious for particular regions than it was prior to the era of agricultural technology. In 1980 the United Nations Food and Agriculture Organization reported famine as a social and physical danger for many of the world's poorest subregions.

Unemployment is another consequence of excessive population growth. The technologies of manufacturing and information processing have reduced labor needs to the point that in the industrialized world (and increasingly in the agrarian world) large families have become economic liabilities instead of assets. Opportunities for personally meaningful, unskilled or manual employment—including farm labor—have diminished. Satisfying work and economic achievement in the technological era are decreasingly available routes to self-affirmation for young men in many parts of the world. The resulting impasse has potentially devastating psychosocial consequences for the next generation: sexual intercourse and reproduction remain routes to self-esteem and personal dignity even as opportunities diminish to become an economically viable father and family provider, a source of both emotional and material support for mate and children. For women, too, having children is a source of self-fulfillment when alternate routes fail to develop.

Children born to poor families, both in the developing world and in the slums of industrialized nations, have overwhelmed public services. Although the health needs of these children are often unmet, public health measures require their physical survival. They survive without benefit of the education essential to their social, economic, and political development and the full expression of their potential as persons. They live in settings that, like the *favelas* of Rio de Janeiro (Brody, 1973), lack community organization and a sense of belonging to any mutual support group outside the immediate family. There, deteriorating settlement patterns and changes in economic opportunity contribute to new and shifting family structures and relationships between the sexes, between generations, and between parents and children. Old people in these settings, alive because of communicable disease control and emergency hospital facilities, lead socially marginal lives and may be victimized by the young. People born into them are often poorly socialized and, as members of excluded or minority groups without access to social power, are not enculturated into the larger society; they have few opportunities to interact with each other and with responsible adults on the basis of common social values. Only the values essential for individual survival (perhaps at the expense of others) are reinforced. Children reared in these settings must attend very early to staying alive and to concrete problem solving. It seems likely that they do not have adequate opportunities for the development of affective sensitivity necessary to the elaboration of empathy, love, guilt, shame—or the wish to achieve that comes from identification with a significant parent of the same sex.

Even in Baltimore, not far from the capital of the United States, changes in birthrate, ethnic status, conjugal relationships, family structure, and economic opportunity seem linked. In a city of under one million inhabitants, 57 percent black and 43 percent white according to the 1980 census, the unemployment rate among young black men approaches 50 percent. From 1963 through 1978 the estimated proportion of out-of-wedlock births in the city rose from 19.8 to 54.1 percent, with 42 percent of these in 1978 born to mothers aged 19 and under. In that year 72 percent of the births to nonwhite city residents were out-of-wedlock, compared with 20 percent of the white births. These differences in reproductive behavior between inner city blacks and whites cannot be accounted for by differences in income level or education alone (Zelnick and Kantner, 1978), but seem to imply cultural differences as well. Similar differences do not exist between black and white middle-class groups in the surrounding suburbs.

The reproductive crisis significantly involves adolescents. Approximately one million women aged 19 or under become pregnant each year in the United States. Approximately 560,000 of these carry their children to term, 330,000 have an abortion, and the rest have spontaneous abortions or miscarriages (National Center for Health Statistics, 1979). The psychosocial risks for adolescent parents and the potential hazards for their offspring are well known. Early childbearing is associated with a lower level of educational achievement for the parents, independent of race or socioeconomic status (Moore and Waite, 1977). This effect is permanent, in that adolescent mothers never achieve the same education as peers who delay parenthood. The age of a high school student's first delivery correlates directly with the amount of schooling she finally completes (Card and Wise, 1978). Adults who were adolescent mothers have lower-status jobs, lower incomes, and less job satisfaction. Disruption of formal education is associated not only with less vocational achievement but also with a higher rate of repeated pregnancy (Klerman and Jekel, 1973; Furstenberg, 1976).

Adolescent fathers have not been so extensively studied, but their difficulties appear comparable in many ways (Elster and McAnarney, 1980). Economic disadvantages are especially prevalent among adolescent boys forced to support a family and to take jobs with less chance of ultimate advancement in order to gain immediate rewards (Furstenberg, 1976; Trussell, 1976).

Concern that the infant of an adolescent parent may not receive adequate care derives from the likelihood that the parent's emotional development is not yet complete. The increased risk among adolescent mothers of having underweight, premature, and stillborn infants or infants who die soon after birth (Menken, 1980) appears to be due mainly to inadequate prenatal care (Baldwin and Cain, 1980). Analyses of all available data from several research projects conducted under the auspices of the National Institute of Health's Center for Population Research (Baldwin and Cain, 1980) also reveal significant risks even for infants who are healthy at birth. These risks, which include deficits in cognitive development, social and emotional development, and school adjustment, are largely associated with the social and economic consequences of early childbearing for the new parents. The children of these adolescents are more likely than those born to older people to spend part of their childhood in one-parent households: the adolescent mother rears her child with help from neither its father nor her own parents.

Studies supported by the Center for Population Research also show that children of adolescent parents are more likely than others to repeat the pattern in their own lives. The human reproductive crisis includes significant intergenerational components. Early sexual intercourse without contraception, followed by pregnancy, delivery, and single-handed rearing of the new infant by an adolescent mother (sometimes with the help of her own mother), seems to constitute a definable behavioral pattern. To the degree that this pattern follows a socially inherited design for living (cf. Kluckhohn, 1944), it may be regarded as an aspect of culture.

The human reproductive crisis, then, is not confined to the massive increase in the number of human beings on the planet. It also refers to the increase in the number of those who are unintended, unwanted, unplanned for, uncared for, and ultimately deprived of chances for optimal development. These people have few chances for adequate parenting or socialization into their communities. The reproductive crisis concerns mature parents burdened with children for whom they cannot or will not care and adolescent parents whose life chances are foreclosed by premature reproduction. It concerns dehumanization to the degree that it deprives people of necessary social experience. It is significant for social evolution to the degree that it is self-perpetuating and will influence the lives of future generations.

One rational solution and preventive for this crisis has been birth control. When the provision of birth control methods and public pressure for their use has come from governments, it has been called population policy. United Nations declarations still urge member states to promote family planning programs (World Health Assembly, 1979), but their statements clearly reveal the ambivalence and sensitivity of governments to fertility issues. One, while declaring that reproduction is a human right, notes that family planning "frees man to attain his individual dignity and reach his full potential." It also reaffirms "the right of couples to determine the number and spacing of their children freely," but specifies that this should be done "responsibly," emphasizing "the right of persons to have access to the relevant information, means and methods for implementation of such decisions" (UN, 1969).

The World Health Organization similarly fails to reconcile the contradictions inherent in the concepts of reproductive freedom and constraint. Family planning, it states, is a "way of thinking and living that is adopted *voluntarily* . . . by individuals and couples" (WHO, 1973). Planning, then, implies limitations; but there is no mention of the alternative—freedom to reproduce to the extent that nature permits. A United Nations symposium in January 1974 came closest to the issue when it referred to "the necessity of defining the scope of this right [to procreate] as well as the right not to procreate." Thus, public opinion is moving slowly and indirectly away from the idea that unlimited reproduction is a universal human right, despite the fact that in August 1974 most Third World nations at the World Population Conference rejected the idea that population growth should be controlled by direct governmental action. They regarded population control as secondary to the achievement of justice, defined mainly in terms of their freedom of economic opportunity vis-à-vis the developed world.

When birth control advice and service has come from agencies and institutions concerned with the quality of life for parents, children, and families, it has been called family planning. When it refers to the capacity of a man or woman to manage his or her own fertility, as an aspect of individual autonomy, it has been called personal fertility regulation. This rational solution has not worked for large segments of the world's people. The technology has been available but it either has not been used or has not, despite instruction and availability, been used competently.

This book examines why contraceptive services have not been adequately used in one small part of the world, Jamaica, viewing its problems in the context of the global reproductive crisis.

Jamaica as a Study Site

Jamaica is an especially interesting and accessible natural laboratory in which to study sexual intercourse as an aspect of human relating, and its reproductive consequences. A small island, its boundaries are self-contained. In 1951 the birthrate in Jamaica was reported as 34.6 per 1,000 women from ages 15 to 44. By 1960 the rate had increased to 42 per 1,000. After that there was a gradual decline, the sharpest drop, from 38.9 to 34.2, occurring in 1966-1968. During 1967-68 the government established a highly visible, intensive program aimed at limiting family size. In 1969 the birthrate was 33 per 1,000 and the population was growing by 2.4 percent yearly. It was predicted in the 1960s that if the birthrate were not reduced to approximately 26 per 1,000, by 1975 the economy would collapse (Walsh, 1970). In 1972 the birthrate was still close to 34 per 1,000 despite the fact that, as one critic of the United States Agency for International Development said, "We have sent them enough condoms to sink the island." As another said, "The biggest export of Jamaica is still Jamaicans."

The birthrate remained between 33 and 34 between 1972 and 1975 during the period of research reported here. In 1973 George Roberts, the island's leading demographer, wrote: "In terms of gross reproduction rates, which are determined essentially by the size and composition of the population within the age span 15-44, there has been no change since 1960" (p. 3). He attributed the recorded decreases to the emigration of 291,000 people between 1960 and 1970, equivalent to more than half the natural increase, including 6 percent of the males and 9 percent of the females between ages 25 and 49. The unaltered islandwide birthrate, of course, did not rule out the possibility of declines in terms of other measures, such as changes in family size. According to the most recent report of the National Planning Agency (November, 1978), "There is no way of evaluating the success of the family planning programme as data are not collected on the number of persons who are continuous users of F.P. methods . . . The number of new acceptors . . . continues at a high rate for the island, but has shown signs of falling off" in the Kingston metropolitan region (p. 37). In 1980 no new birthrate data were available.

The government's inability to manage the fertility of its citizens stimulated considerable research during the period before 1967-1968 when the systematic program of family planning was initiated. Books by Blake (1961), Stycos and Back (1964), and Smith (1962) explored these issues. They and especially Edith Clarke (1957) also recognized the striking prevalence of mother-headed households and of children reared without the consistent presence of an economically viable father. An earlier work by Kerr (1952) had suggested a negative overall impact of the social system and family structure on the personality of children.

Besides its high birthrate, Jamaica shares many socioeconomic features with other developing countries and with the poverty-stricken backwaters of industrialized nations, especially those with significant ethnic minorities. Its pattern of domestic unions has much in common with those encountered among poor black North Americans. Households with young children tend to be headed by women who have produced children by more than one man. Maternal grandmothers are important culture figures. First pregnancy typically occurs during adolescence, with the infant turned over to the young mother's own mother. The more important the maternal grandmother and the younger or less economically viable the father, the more peripheral he is in the early lives of his children. Relatively few Jamaican mothers have the security of marriage when their babies are small.

Lack of education is another common factor in developing countries and in the impoverished areas of industrialized nations. Like most people distant from the sources of societal power, the majority of Jamaicans, including many with the largest families, have not gone beyond primary school. They feel little or no identification with modern scientific and technological values and with national population policy. Profertility values exist in many folk beliefs and attitudes. A woman, for example, has a foreordained "lot" of babies; if she does not have the full allotted number she may fall ill. One who has not produced a baby in some inland parishes by age 15 is called a mule, a sterile freak of nature. Contraceptives are dangerous for a variety of reasons: the condom will "fly up into the shoulder"; the IUD will "suck you down." The government family planning program and the methods it advocates are designated by colloquial terms with repressive or unnatural connotations, such as "the planning" or "the control."

Jamaican society is rich in supernatural figures, with whom contact is maintained through a variety of mediums and healers. Yet Jamaicans are aware of and appreciate their medical school, hospitals, private physicians, and public clinics. Even elderly people from inland parishes say that no one depends totally upon folk or religious healers; they "look for the doctor" if they have "really serious" or potentially incapacitating problems persisting after an initial consultation with a healer or attributable to actual "disease" or injury. In Kingston easy access to medical centers encourages attendance by those who would otherwise ignore their discomfort, treat themselves or their children with home remedies, or seek help from healers.

Jamaica also resembles other developing countries in the youth of its population. The majority of Jamaicans are age 15 or under. The visitor to Kingston is impressed by the number of young children in the "yards" and by the number of youths on the city streets. Poor, slum-dwelling parents, especially mothers who are household heads, express bittersweet feelings about their large families. They love their children, and their sons and daughters mean a great deal to them. At the same time, they are painfully aware of their inability to educate, shelter, clothe, or even feed them as they would like. Despite occasional efforts at self-deception, they know that their offspring's chances for a decent life may be limited. Despite the socially and culturally supported value of children, the high status of parenthood in Jamaica, and their apprehension about putting modern contraceptive devices or chemicals into their bodies, they are aware of the advantages of personal fertility control. At the same time, they are in conflict about engaging in it. Even with mixed feelings and regrets, they continue to reproduce under circumstances militating against optimum development for themselves as parents and adults, for their children as future adults, and for all as members of a family desiring the best life possible.

The Development of Family Planning Services in Jamaica

The island's rapid population increase, the result of a continuing high birthrate and declining levels of infant mortality, has been regarded as a national problem by government planners and leading citizens since at least 1940. Most recently concern has focused on the quality of life and potential competence of children born to parents without the resources to care properly for them and those in family units without a consistent, stable, economically or emotionally supportive father. The transfer of responsibility for child care, referred to as "passing on," with abandonment as its ultimate expression, has been "developed to a fine point in this culture" (Brodber, 1974, p. 49). Brodber regards the neglect by biological parents of their children's sleeping or eating as well as total health as especially widespread in the Kingston slum yards.

These social concerns have political and economic roots. In 1938 a strike at the West Indies Sugar Company led to a series of riots during which several laborers were killed by police and many more injured. Disorders in Kingston and elsewhere provided an organizing focus for both the class-linked fears and the developing social conscience of educated Jamaicans. A direct consequence was the formation in Kingston in 1939 of the Jamaican Birth Control League, which in 1941 became the Jamaica Family Planning League. In 1950 the first family planning services were offered in St. Ann, a small community on the north shore of the island, as part of a child welfare clinic. Despite public attacks, the work proceeded with the active support and collaboration of socially motivated citizens, including nurses and physicians. Demand grew so rapidly that a new agency was founded. Other clinics slowly developed and in 1957 all were united in the Jamaica Family Planning Association (JFPA), affiliated with the International Planned Parenthood Federation. As acceptance developed, the Child Welfare Association of Jamaica in 1961 included family planning as part of its program. The central Kingston clinic on East Street began operating in 1962, the year of Jamaica's official independence from Great Britain.

A policy statement incorporated in the national Five Year Plan for 1963-1968 resolved to "bring about a greater awareness of the implications of rapid population growth and population pressure in the island . . . as well as the effects of excessive childbearing on the lives and prospects of individuals. [The government] will encourage the spread of information on and techniques for the spacing or limitation of families for the benefit of those persons who desire them."

By 1965 a Family Planning Unit was established in the Ministry of Health. This was superseded in 1967 by the National Family Planning Board (NFPB), and in late 1970 legislation made the board a legal entity. Government planners concluded that it was not feasible to await the attainment of preconditions—expected to be industrialization, education, literacy, a middle class, acceptance of modern values—for lowered death rates followed by reduced fertility rates. National fertility was making it impossible for new schools and job opportunities to catch up with the growing population.

Geographic accessibility does not seem to be the major factor determining contraceptive use or nonuse. Since 1968 the government has blanketed the island with billboards, radio and television announcements, newspaper advertisements, and family planning clinics. No Jamaican lives more than six miles from a clinic (Sinclair, 1974). Between 1972 and 1975, the period of this study, there were 162 government or JFPA family planning clinics in the country, including 5 open daily and 33 with scheduled sessions during the week in the Kingston Metropolitan Area. Three others were local satellites of major clinics (Statistical Report, NFPB, 1974). The JFPA East Street clinic was the single major nonhospital family planning facility in the Kingston Metropolitan Area and the best-known source of contraceptive services.

National Family Planning Board data from the second quarter of 1974 indicate the status of clinical operations during this study. In this quarter 5,811 new acceptors of family planning were registered along with 45,830 revisits. In Kingston new acceptors seemed to be decreasing, an impression confirmed in 1978 by the National Planning Agency. At the East Street clinic, for example, there were 295 new acceptors for the second quarter of 1974, compared with a quarterly average of 329 in 1972 and 437 in 1971. The declining age of new acceptors suggests that the majority of interested, older, residentially stable women might have already visited the clinic and that the new acceptors were largely young recent migrants from rural areas. Despite the apparent increase in new acceptors in the rest of the island in 1978, especially among younger women, the lack of a major decline in the overall birthrate suggests that they are inconsistent or inefficient in their subsequent use of the methods.

The one systematically controlled study of the introduction of contraceptive opportunity into a Jamaican community showed that it had no demonstrable effect (K. A. Smith, 1971). Although a high proportion of potential users said they would use planning services should these become available, a very small proportion actually used the service when it was initiated and only a fraction of these maintained any consistent effective contact over the 40-month period of the study. Nor was there a significant difference in recruitment to family planning services between a community that offered an educational program and services and a control community that remained untreated. The problem seemed to be not physical but psychosocial accessibility. Understanding the psychosocial barriers to contraceptive use means understanding how Kingston men and women feel and think and what they do about managing their own fertility. This requires studying how they feel, think, and act about sexual intercourse with or without contraception; about living, loving, and relating with each other; about becoming parents or not; and about having few or many children. The interdependence of personal biography, sociocultural context, and fertility-related behavior, including individual efforts to modify it in oneself, has not been studied since the advent of easily available, technically effective contraceptive methods. This book presents the results of such a study.

2　An Approach to the Problem: Epistemological Aspects of Interviewing and Clinical Practice in the Field

How can an investigator comprehend a people's feelings and decisions about their own fertility? Are observations by an outsider relevant to the subjective experience of individual insiders? Understanding through combined participation and observation stems in part from the investigator's struggle for acceptance, the adaptive effort to establish a new equilibrium in strange surroundings, and the attempt to perceive life in the way that those in the new community do.

The information acquired from a research subject through systematic interviews constitutes a kind of cultural map of the new context, influenced by the personal characteristics of the informant and the evolution of the informant-ethnographer relationship. This cultural map cannot logically correspond to, or represent an identity with, so-called facts existing "out there," in the objective world. Instead it serves as a basis on which the ethnographer—in this instance the student of sexual-reproductive behavior patterns—will create a construct: an account of the sexual-reproductive aspects of a culture, including the role of parenting. At its best, such a construct organizes a range of disparate observations, providing coherence and maximum correspondence among phenomena revealed through different techniques, subjects, or investigators.

Clues to a culture, a group's socially inherited design for living (Kluckhohn, 1944), are identifiable in specific interactions between individuals. These include sexual interactions that may or may not be intended or allowed to have reproductive consequences. Edward Sapir noted that the locus of culture may also be found "in the world of meanings which each one . . . may unconsciously abstract for himself from his participation in these interactions" (1932, p. 236). Patterns of sexual-reproductive behavior, for example, cannot be understood without reference to their meanings for the individuals who engage in them. These may be idiosyncratic and determined by individual biography. At the same time they are functions of the knowledge, psychological states, attitudes, and values common to (most of) the population involved that constitute, in Linton's term, the "covert" aspects of a culture (1945). Its "overt" aspects are the actual behaviors that most people in the society engage in throughout their life cycle. To the degree that individuals consistently and systematically relate the publicly observable surface to what is private, "deep," or covert, the congruence may be designated as a collective pattern. This study is concerned with collective patterns of reproductive behavior and the impact of a government population policy upon them.

Most students, considering the survival value of social organization, have approached human fertility from the viewpoint of society. They have dealt mainly with decision making, risk taking, the value of children, family size preferences, and the construction of economic utility models of childbearing. Some research has been essentially demographic. Other studies, viewing reproductive behavior as a cultural issue, have considered such matters as indigenous fertility-regulating methods—those occurring "naturally" in a community—and the acceptability to particular populations of technological methods introduced by governments or social agencies (Newman, 1980). This study is concerned with the acceptance of technological fertility-regulating methods originating in the industrially developed world by members of a society that is still undergoing industrialization. Investigation of the topic involves considering the ways in which social structure influences patterns of sexual relating, overt or covert reproductive decisions, how they are acted upon, and their consequences. It also deals with the way in which technological methods are presented to the public—under what circumstances, and by whom. The acceptability of an unfamiliar method of regulating a valued psychosocial and biological function often depends on the potential user's relations with the individual or group providing the method.

This study is concerned also with the symbolic significance of sex and reproduction and the values attached to them, their personal and social antecedents and consequences, and the consequences and meaning of limiting one's potential fertility in a particular community. Knowledge of these matters is essential to understanding the way in which family planning services are received. Beyond this point, sexual-reproductive behavior is private, burdened with intrapsychic as well as interpersonal conflicts, and evocative of personal security operations. It involves relationships between people who have sexual intercourse together and either do or do not anticipate the possible reproductive consequences of their acts. "Couple communication" is determined both by social structure and by culture.

Based on this approach, the investigator's task involves learning about the private and individual as well as public and shared meanings of having children, increasing or limiting the size of one's family, letting nature take its sexual-reproductive course, or examining and managing the possible reproductive consequences of one's sexual acts and relationships. It also involves learning about both the covert and overt aspects of reproductively significant interactions. Systematic interviewing can accomplish part of this task. Participating both in the life of the community and in clinical interaction fills another important requirement. Most significant is the investigator's responsible, personal act of comprehension. The personal quality of this comprehension is "objective in the sense of establishing contact with a hidden reality . . . the condition for anticipating an indeterminate range of . . . true implications" (Polanyi, 1958, pp. vii–viii).

The Role of the Participant-Observer

The investigator in a foreign society has a special identity in terms of social role and function. The patients and staff at the

University of the West Indies (UWI) Department of Psychiatry, where I worked as a visiting professor and consultant, knew me as a psychoanalytically trained psychiatrist. The staff at the Jamaica Family Planning Association (JFPA) and at the Edna Manley Comprehensive Health Clinic, where two colleagues and I interviewed respondents for the study, knew I was a psychiatrist but identified me mainly as a physician. The clients or patients at these two agencies knew me as a physician who was, unlike them, white and a foreigner, American or English. (The difference in my nationality was not always apparent to them, and for most it seemed unimportant.)

The role of the physician is universally recognized. It simultaneously permits contact and sets certain limits upon intimacy. The patient confides in the physician in the knowledge that these revelations will be helpful for both. Medical knowledge depends upon the activity of intervention in a world "reconstituted or transformed in actuality by human practice" (Wartofsky, 1977, p. 170). It is knowledge for some good, value bound, with immediate consequences for human life.

My knowledge of patients at UWI came through clinical interaction in the psychiatric clinic, wards, and the Casualty Department, where emergency cases came, as well as from patients in the care of the WHO psychiatrist attached to the Jamaican government in the hospital and clinic at Savannah-la-Mar or of staff members at the Belleview public mental hospital. At JFPA and Manley it came from research interviews, but in every instance clients or patients were free to ask my advice or that of my two Jamaican psychiatrist colleagues, who conducted the bulk of the interviews; most expressed pleasure at the opportunity to talk about themselves. In these contexts knowledge came from the activity called practicing medicine.

My knowledge also came in part from interacting with members of the society as part of my adaptation to the new environment. Being a participant-observer requires both "involvement and detachment." The investigator's self-image is "stepping in and stepping out" of a society (Powdermaker, 1966, p. 290). Robert Murphy (1971, p. 11) implied the problems of simultaneous incompatible goals requiring personal involvement when he wrote of "converting ourselves into instruments while struggling to maintain our identities." There is an intrapsychic tension associated with getting to know and identify with one's new neighbors as friends or colleagues and at the same time using them as sources of information, which requires distancing and objectifying. Depending on personal characteristics and activities, the investigator—regardless of professional role—will eventually be assigned a role, a social identity, in the new community.

As a physician I was recognized as offering a service that legitimated my entry into the new community. At the University I was invited to provide a medical teaching service, in which I had to function as an active diagnostician/therapist. The clinician-ethnographer in this mold is an intentional intervener, invited by members of the community to use the power of person, foreign ideas, and technology in a situation demanding change. Studying reproduction, and especially family planning, was not compatible with that role. It was one I established for myself, and in doing so aroused some potential doubts among colleagues who were sensitive to culturally inappropriate, perhaps even colonialist, attitudes about limiting the fertility of Jamaicans with techniques imported from North America or the United Kingdom. These colleagues tended to identify me with the family planning cause.

For patients and clients, however, there seemed no such doubts. They recognized that to perform a therapeutic service, an officially designated healer requires access to their minds and bodies. Turning to a physician, even a foreign one, seemed to be a natural response to anticipated or actual pain, disability (including unwanted pregnancy), or impending death. Those who sought such help were highly motivated informants, expecting the clinician to do something about their problem. The seeker's perception occurs in a context in which the healer's commitment is mutual. This structure of expectations is an aspect of the social contract. In the clinical interaction—including psychotherapy with upper-class Jamaicans—I experienced none of the occasional uneasiness that emerged from time to time in close conversation with medical colleagues or new acquaintances in Kingston's active and widely traveled group of professional intellectuals. With them the medical role was no protection from my having to struggle for acceptance as a person. In contrast, with patients the medical role provided a comforting sense of beneficial exchange: their cultural information in return for my medical assistance. The familiar activities of diagnosing and treating were at times clearly insulating from problematic aspects of the new setting, as well as reassuring in their affirmation of a familiar identity and sense of being a continuing entity despite diminished customary feedback. The protection which the clinical relationship offers the doctor depends in part upon its being bounded and in many ways ritualized. In contrast, there is a continuing real life engagement, without role boundaries, with influential people and friends who become informants in the new community. They hold actual power over the investigator, who despite his or her social status is a supplicant in search of hidden cultural knowledge (Brody and Newman, 1981).

It was perhaps for this reason that my moments of greatest personal freedom occurred in social interactions with members of the small group of expatriates living in Kingston. No culture includes among its available roles that of an object of study for a person from another culture. With the expatriate group there was no risk of threatening their status as autonomous observers, and this may have afforded us all a certain relaxation, freedom from the need to observe and from concern about being observed. I experienced similar relaxation with a few Jamaican friends whom I met through the expatriates and who were not professional intellectuals or associated with the medical or university establishments. It quickly became apparent, however, that attitudes about sex and reproduction among these relatively affluent and educated Jamaicans resembled those among my research informants. Thus, one day a week was accepted as the man's night out, and on these occasions some of the people I knew were able to attend parties, dine in restaurants, or go dancing with sexual partners whom they ordinarily saw only in private or during the day. My male friends valued their potency highly, made sure they were not too tired on nights when they were with girl friends, and risked no chance of being sexually incompetent. Upper- and lower-class women alike deplored childlessness and expressed pity for friends who were "barren" and had "no one for" their "old age." While some men revealed "outside" children, most, however—unlike those of lower socioeconomic status —did not want children whom they would not rear themselves. The data about male contraceptive users reported in the following chapters also suggest that attitudes revealed in conversation with upper-class men do not predict their actual contraceptive-reproductive behavior.

During my stay in Jamaica I also made some home visits, almost unheard of for one with the status of a professor. Some colleagues wondered why I should leave the company of my peers for the unknown risks and implied pleasures of the town. They also identified my being a white, middle-aged male from a dominant society as factors that could influence my interaction with others, and regarded my size, greater than that of most Jamaicans, as a source of security for me in presumably dangerous neighborhoods. It may have been another indication of their perceived difference between myself and the people with whom I talked. Late in 1973 a senior colleague with whom I was by then on close terms declared, "If you can't grow a black skin you might at least put some hair on your face!" I returned to the island after the Christmas vacation with a mustache. One colleague in the department laughed when she saw me: "Oh, Professor, you used to be a nice doctor, but now you are a man!" On New Year's Eve of 1973, moving from home to home with one of my students, I had a sense of his Kingston world. Later, in the Ethiopian church, I recognized another Kingston world. It was only in retrospect that I understood that the various social worlds of Kingston, easily differentiated in terms of social class, are in fact part of the same historical-cultural matrix. These were among the elements contributing to my experience for approximately eleven months of residence in Kingston—and more than three years of dealing with that experience both on the island and off—between February 1, 1972 and the end of April 1975.

The Person of the Participant-Observer

It was raw and cold on the February morning when I first left Baltimore for Jamaica, but as coats and sweaters were stowed

The task formulated by WHO and the university was to organize a course for registrars (the equivalent of United States hospital residents) in psychotherapy, aimed at qualifying them for the British diploma in psychological medicine.

Although I was delighted with the invitation, remembering the prevalent psychosocial problems of deprived people in Rio and Baltimore I wondered about the task: self-realization can be illusory for people who find it difficult even to conceive of self-determination. I began to inquire about the island as a social setting and the ways in which the place might mold the people who grow up there. Beaubrun also had evidently thought about this, for not long after our talk he sent me a book by Rex M. Nettleford, *Mirror, Mirror: Identity, Race and Protest in Jamaica*. The "trinity of identity, race and protest," Nettleford wrote in 1970, mirrors important aspects of the young nation's major dilemma (p. 9). Whereas "in the contemporary United States racial tension can be said to be a prime reason why poverty has become a major issue, in Jamaica poverty has been a major reason why race-and-colour . . . has become a primary issue" (p. 11).

The book directed my attention to a host of related problems, but one seized my interest above all others. It was the birthrate that made it difficult for many poor Jamaicans to care adequately for their families, and threatened to overwhelm the island's resources.

Jamaica's "population problem" became my immediate choice as a research topic for several other reasons, one of them based in my own early history. I was still a child when I began to realize, through the writings and conversation of my father, a professional scientist, that we humans inhabit a finite planet and our resources are limited. When the notion of "spaceship earth" became popular many years later, it seemed merely a public announcement of what I had known all my life. I also knew early that more advanced species, like microbial colonies, could grow, expand, reach the limits of their development, recede, and die. Then, when I was in my teens, my father first entered the arena of social problems. In an address to a society of biological scientists he pointed to the limited food and energy resources of our globe and advocated the systematic encouragement of birth control. This speech, delivered in the 1930s, evoked an outpouring of hostile letters that puzzled, distressed, and sometimes angered my father. He felt that people should have the right to manage their own fertility as a means of giving their children an optimum chance at life, and that their governments owed them this right. He felt that those who wrote the letters attacking him and his proposals, often on grounds of immorality, were deceiving themselves because they could not confront the disturbing truth. Above all, he thought that persons who wished to control their own fertility should be able to do so.

My father continued his research, which had practical implications for food production. It took him to many countries and brought international graduate students to our home. Although I disappointed him by going to medical school instead of getting a Ph.D., I started a lifetime of compensatory fence-straddling by remaining in academic life and doing research as well as treating patients. My most intense interest was the private, unexplicated, interior life of individuals, but I published the required papers dealing with control groups, statistical approximations, and the characteristics of populations. I did, however, after completing my residency in psychiatry, commute from New Haven to New York for psychoanalytic training.

In 1957, having finished my work with the New York Psychoanalytic Institute, I left the Yale faculty to join the University of Maryland. The episode concerning birth control in the 1930s was long forgotten, but it reemerged unexpectedly late in 1967 or early in 1968. En route to Lima for a meeting with South American colleagues, I talked with Dr. Henry David, a psychologist, recently of the Geneva office of the World Federation of Mental Health, which was also meeting in Lima. David was in the process of establishing a series of research projects in family planning in several European and Asian countries. During the next three years I accompanied him as a psychiatric consultant to projects in Prague and Budapest and a joint meeting of the WHO sections of Mental Health and Human Reproduction in Geneva. As a result, when I arrived in Jamaica I was ready to become interested in its human and social problems associated with large families and rapid population growth. It was almost inevitable, as well, that I should continue to struggle to reconcile my simultaneous interest in individuals and in populations.

This personal background is related to the epistemological problems of this kind of research, which I regard as one approach to the classic problem of other minds. We come to know other people and the contexts of their lives by living, working, and talking intimately with them. No observation is untouched by the influence of the observer. This is especially true when the objects of knowledge are fellow human beings. The observer registers what is happening with his feelings, thoughts, and perceptions shaped by previous experience. The more intimate the study, the more the participants in the encounter constitute a unit. A patient revealing himself to an inquiring and listening psychoanalyst who responds in turn, is less object than subject. The listener's access to the patient's psychological interior is determined by his introspective-empathic capacity, which includes intimate access to his own mind.

First Contact: The Doctor-Patient Relationship

The patients whom I encountered at the UWI Hospital were mainly poor, underemployed, and semiliterate; many believed in magic or folk healing. They were treated by people who, while sharing their West Indian origins, belonged to a different social class. The doctors, often educated in Scotland or England, were from economically comfortable families. Their deeply ingrained paternalistic attitudes reinforced the patients' postures of dependency and supplication. Although color was not identified as an issue, patients were more often black and doctors brown. As a result of my "objective" observations, my background as a student of culture in relation to behavior, and my initial loneliness and need for communication in the new environment, I soon concluded that the training in psychoanalytic psychotherapy that was my official mission was inappropriate for the needs of either group. It seemed to me that the patients needed an advocate and that the doctors should, simply, direct their patients less and listen to them more. I felt that ordinary, everyday communication, including the sharing of feelings, was more needed than training in the technical aspects of psychotherapy.

The doctors, whose training had emphasized the rapid and massive use of tranquillizing drugs and electroshock therapy and who spoke with authority as native West Indians, felt that this change in approach would be a grave mistake. They believed that the patients expected unambiguous direction and advice, whether from Western or local healers, and that they required concrete, "strong" medicine, by mouth or by injection. They were more interested in acquiring new technical procedures that would increase their professional status.

Under these circumstances, feeling isolated both from my ordinary interpersonal network and from my professional subculture, I decided that the quickest way to get my bearings would be to immerse myself in hospital life, particularly that of the emergency or Casualty Department. It was important, though, to recognize that the opportunity to care for others could be used to deal with my unconscious feeling of abandonment in a way that might impair the accuracy of my observations.

On my second evening in Kingston the registrar on call was busy, so the nurse asked me to see a patient, who she said had had a manic episode but now seemed quiet enough to be admitted for investigation of a presumed ulcer. The chart contained a brief description of her reason for admission: epigastric discomfort several hours after meals, relieved by milk. Then there was an account of acute, violent agitation and assaultive behavior requiring restraint by several aides and the intramuscular injection of thorazine.

I found the patient, a woman looking at least ten years older than her stated age of 47, with black skin and rather thin graying hair, lying on top of a narrow bed in a corner of the large open room. She was dressed in a worn hospital robe. A paper shopping bag was on the floor between her and the wall, and on the bedside table was a can containing earth in which grew a single flower. After a slow start she became animated and our conversation lasted for almost two hours, interrupted by tea that I brought from the nurse's station. She had brought her flower from home, a shanty community along Spanishtown Road. She had several children, including grown daughters with children of their own, but now lived alone without a regular man, although there was one who visited from time to time and occasionally gave her some money. She had brought the flower, she said, simply because she wanted something familiar with her, never having been in a hospital before. When the nurse had tried to remove it, saying dirt would be spilled on the table, the patient had protested so vehemently that the nurse sent an aide to administer a sedative tablet. But the patient was unaccustomed to swallowing pills, she said, and anyway her throat was dry, so she asked for a glass of water. The aide paid no attention and simply placed the pill in her mouth. When the patient spat it out, the aide seemed to take it personally and wouldn't talk with her any more. Instead she brought two men who grabbed her arms and legs, turned her over, and gave her a painful injection in her buttocks. At some point in our exchange, which involved her identifying me as a visiting World Health Organization doctor from the United States and still a stranger on the island, she asked me to have a look at her buttocks, which I did. There was a puncture mark on each, with still swollen surrounding areas confirming forceful jabs with a needle into noncooperative flesh.

It is evident that my perceived status facilitated and shaped the nature of the patient's account. Furthermore, my identification with her, of which I became aware only the next morning, influenced not only the manner in which I elicited her story but also my evaluation of what she had to say. That morning I awakened in my room at the Mona Hotel, an old Jamaican greathouse on beautiful grounds, still used by a generation of elderly guests from Great Britain, many of whom had once lived on the island. As my eye registered the luxuriant bougainvillea outside my window, I remembered the single flower in the scrubby can cherished by last night's patient, and also, fleetingly, a dream of having been in a garden. Having been trained to pay attention to my own dreams as well as those of my patients, it did not take long to follow my associations back to the garden of my childhood home; to confront my transitory wishes while in foreign countries to be back in familiar surroundings; to recall my momentary despair at the age of nine on my first day in a Parisian public school, when I realized that I could not speak French and no one there could really speak English; and via a series of more intimate associations to grasp my sense of fellowship and identity with the patient as though we were both persecuted strangers, misunderstood in an alien land. I also remembered that an analyst's dream about a patient indicates a countertransference process—the development of feelings, attitudes, or ideas with roots in the unresolved or reactivated conflicts of the analyst's own past—and that this process distorts his perception of so-called objective reality. That is, it influences the process of psychoanalytic knowing.

In this instance my dream enhanced my wish to keep in touch with the patient. She was my initial window to the medical culture of the island as experienced by the poor. I saw her twice more while she was hospitalized having x-ray studies. These proved diagnostically negative, but along with whatever else was going on seemed to result in at least temporary disappearance of her symptoms. She returned twice at one-week intervals to see me in my office. Two things became quickly apparent: first, that she had a special regard for me, not so much because I was different and outside the system in which she felt trapped, but because of the time I gave her and my evident willingness to listen; and second, that she was a suspicious and isolated person, though not one whom I could fit into a psychiatric category, perhaps because my perception was clouded by my initial identification with her. Her world view included two institutions that could be simultaneously helpful and dangerous. One was Obeah, the type of West African sorcery transplanted to the Caribbean; she spoke of an Obeahman along the Spanishtown Road whom she consulted for a variety of physical discomforts but who she later thought might have been responsible for some of them. The other was the hospital where she finally went, feeling that it might provide not only relief for bodily symptoms but also protection against a possible Obeah spell. I began to realize, especially as we talked about the various men who had fathered her children—in her terms, "for whom" she had had babies—that she used me, like the Obeahman, as a combined person and social institution. She was struggling to resolve conflicting perceptions of me as a nurturing and potentially dangerous parent and also as a man, who like any other man could become a sexual partner, the father of her child, and later—like her actual partner—leave her alone. Her early ambivalence toward authority embodied in males had developed in a matrifocal family and contributed to her private use of these public symbols of helping and dangerous powers.

In the course of these talks I learned that she had not "seen her period" for almost two years and had wondered for part of this time if she might be pregnant. Now, having had sexual intercourse only rarely, the last time three months earlier with the visiting man who left her some money, she thought she might be going through the change of life. The plant that she had brought to keep her company and probably represented home and security—and in terms of our retrospective exploration, her childhood with her mother high in the St. Andrew hills—was a marigold. I learned from her and later confirmed elsewhere that the marigold was known for "bringing down the period when it not seen for a while."

The flower, the central focus of our brief series of interviews, emerged with several simultaneous meanings.

It became a unifier with joint biographical meaning, for in the interest of reducing her isolation and increasing her sense of personal worth I shared my dream with her. Moreover, beginning with the cultural significance of the marigold as a symbol of fertility—pregnancy incurred but not wished for, or menses disappeared and brought back—we were able to associate her rage at being imposed upon in the hospital with her anger at nonsupportive and exploiting males and with her sense of loss of femaleness as her periods were disappearing permanently: a sharp contrast with the hopefulness of childhood and youth, when she lived in the country nurtured by her mother and surrounded by flowering plants.

I concluded that she was depressed (though not necessarily suffering from a depression) and that her stomach discomfort was an expression of longing, deprivation, and a wish once more to be cared for like a child and valued as a woman. I noted further (1) that my evaluations of her and our interaction were determined by a transference relationship that itself constituted an important part of the data; (2) that cultural forms always have private meaning for the people involved in them; and (3) that the familiar activities of diagnosing and treating behavior were adaptive and security enhancing for me in the new setting.

This was my first contact with the ubiquitous tension between Jamaican men and women about the issues of sex and reproduction. I understood it as a partial function of the context of reproductive behavior. Human behavior at any moment reflects not only the impact of earlier development but also participation in a continuing social process. The relationship between context-related process and private meanings generated during cumulative individual life experience is richly evident in the patterns of feeling, thinking, and acting that collectively constitute reproductive behavior. Comparisons of such behavior between cultures illuminate features that may appear enigmatic within a single context. At the same time, reproductive behavior has certain common features that reflect "general, shared or prevalent qualities of private life" (Levy, 1974, p. xvii). It may also be considered one of those "constants of the human situation" in which a clinically involved investigator might identify "the shared symbolic and interactional contexts through which the individual experiences human universals" (Levine, 1973, p. 248).

Sampling and Interviewing

One route to understanding is through planned conversation, often called interviewing. The question then arises, who is to be interviewed? Demographers and epidemiologists are especially concerned that a sample population be sufficiently representative to warrant its use as the basis for generalization. This approach ordinarily requires a group, controlled for age, socioeconomic status, and other factors, interviewed by a worker going from door to door in selected neighborhoods. Randomly selected subjects tend, however, to lack motivation. They also lack the other factors inherent in a potentially significant relationship with a person who wears the cultural mantle of the healer. I tried to reconcile sampling requirements with my wish to obtain the kind of information ordinarily produced by a motivated person speaking to a physician or a helping person in a clinical setting: information that is often concealed from others and sometimes from oneself. I began to ask patients, nonprofessional hospital staff members, market higglers, store clerks, and men next to me at the bar where I occasionally stopped for a Red Stripe beer, about health in relation to "modern values." These conversations were necessarily roundabout and incomplete, but a general tendency was apparent. The person wishing for greater effectiveness—physical strength, sexual potency, more children, success in love or work—would try at first to achieve it independently. Such achievement seemed to depend more often upon a change in diet or a special food or "tea" than upon systematic learning or even exercise. A "natural" substance ingested orally was a preferred means of self-change. If this did not work a "shepherd," Obeahman, or balm-healer might be consulted. Improving oneself and personal fulfillment were not goals for which a physician was consulted. If, on the other hand, "me know something wrong wit' me," the medical doctor came quickly to mind, despite the recognition that "dem' doctors not know all." Once I had a flat tire in a remote section of the West Kingston slum. The young men who, within minutes, surrounded me looked at my beaten-up Volkswagen, my loose tropical shirt identical with their own, and, despite a deep tan, my unequivocal whiteness. Only one type of white man would be driving that kind of car in that neighborhood. One youngster asked almost immediately, "You, doctor from University Hospital?" And upon my affirmative reply several thrust forward with real or made-up complaints, most presented with laughter, as one, opening his mouth, cried, "Hey doc, look at me tongue!" My tire was changed by three or four of the group, working together, and within half an hour I was on my way.

Next, I decided to talk with those entrusted with distributing contraceptive information and supplies, and with some of the people who came to them. During my second month on the island I visited a number of family planning centers. Because of the interested assistance of the staff, the central Jamaica Family Planning Association (JFPA) clinic at 65 East Street in the center of Kingston Parish, the old town, became my headquarters for learning about local family planning and population activities. The clinic staff made it possible for me to conduct a series of long, intensive interviews with women coming for contraceptive advice or materials. On the basis of reading, conversation with staff members, and the interviews I constructed a data recording schedule. With this as a guide I conducted an additional series of intensive, psychodynamically oriented interviews, each about two and a half hours long, with 30 women.

By this time it was clear that contraceptive use and nonuse were issues of sufficient complexity that the interviewing would have to include not only contraceptors but also noncontraceptors and perhaps people in some intermediate category. I determined that the socioeconomic status of JFPA clients was modal for the Kingston area. All were sufficiently comfortable with the official health care system to depend upon it for contraceptive or medical services. It remained uncertain, however, whether there was any association between a positive attitude to modern health care and willingness to use a technical contraceptive device. A continuing relationship with a clinic or physician could indicate comfortable dependence on an available source of nurture and knowledge. On the other hand, a woman willing to swallow a pill or insert a foreign object into her vagina in order to prevent intercourse from resulting in pregnancy could be more active, autonomous, independent, or "modern"; less passive, dependent, or traditional; and in any event less fearful or constrained than one who let nature take its course. This could also be true, though to a lesser degree, for women with partners who assumed responsibility for fertility control by using condoms, in contrast with women whose mates opposed contraception.

In order to obtain a sample of the range of contraceptive use large enough to permit statistical analysis yet small enough to be manageable, I decided to interview 150 women: 50 late users of contraception with three or more children at the time of first consultation with the JFPA; 50 early users with zero to two children at the time of first contact; and 50 nonusers. The 100 users were to be interviewed at the JFPA East Street clinic. After reviewing various available populations, including those at clinics associated with UWI, I selected the Edna Manley Comprehensive Health Clinic, with a population of comparable socioeconomic status, as the site for interviewing the 50 nonusers. Its clinic status would also, it was felt, provide a group comparable to the others in their Western health service orientation. The director of the clinic and her staff made it possible for me to spend several hours daily for a week, observing the diagnosis and treatment activities there and conducting detailed interviews with ten patients. Staff members estimated that "at the most" only every fifth or sixth sexually active female patient at this center was currently using a technical method.

On the basis of all available data and a systematic review of the research literature, I constructed new, more comprehensive data recording schedules. These were used for training the two senior psychiatric registrars who were interested in the project and joined me with the approval of the department director. Another series of interviews was discarded and the data schedule further revised.

As my new colleagues and I gradually came to know and feel more free with one another, we recognized that their attitudes toward patients were more directive than mine, reflecting their own life experience with working-class compatriots—including hospital patients—and their graduate education in the British Isles. The social gulf between the majority of Jamaicans and the educated elite reinforced their tendency to ask short, directive questions. It also reinforced the tendency of patients or family planning clients to respond with brief, conforming answers. After repeated discussion, observation of interviewing technique, and the joint transfer of data from process notes to recording form, we achieved a level of apparent agreement. Later comparison of our notes indicated that we made almost identical judgments about the clients we interviewed; yet we never fully resolved differences in our implicit attitudes toward patients. I tended to see them more as creatures of culture and early life experience. They continued, in keeping with the British psychiatric tradition, to be more impressed by the possible roles of constitution and genetic endowment.

By now we had decided that the interviews should focus on the client's or patient's sexual, contraceptive, conjugal, and childbearing history within an overall biographical context. The manner of interviewing was essentially nondirective. Missed, glossed over, or uncertain points were returned to at the end of the first phase of the interview and reexamined with gentle probing until there was a consensus between subject and interviewer. In order to ensure accuracy, dates, ages when particular events occurred, and ages of children were rechecked with the client before the interview was terminated. Similarly, "don't know" or "all right" responses, suggesting conscious evasion or repression of material easily accessible to consciousness, elicited further attention from the interviewer. After the formal interview respondents were asked to tell a brief story about each of five Thematic Apperception Test pictures that portrayed interaction between figures interpretable as man and woman or parent and child. Each was then asked to draw a person, then a person of the opposite sex, and to say something about them. When women said they did not want to do the drawing, they were invited only once again to do so.

Actual interviewing for data to be retained for statistical analysis began in late 1973, and most of the JFPA clients were seen during 1974. Only one interviewer was present on any one day so as to obtain maximum privacy during interviewing and avoid disruptions of clinic activity. The place was not crowded and, as a rule, few women were awaiting attention. The first to appear after the interviewer's arrival was asked by the nurse in charge if she would be willing to talk with a physician about her reproductive and contraceptive history as part of a research project. Almost none refused, and because those who were employed had invariably been granted a free half-day, all were able to remain for the lengthy interview. Interviews were usually conducted in an office with a closed door excluding most of the sounds of clinic activity.

The interviewers were particularly alert to possible "yea-saying," or automatically giving conforming answers. This was not a persistent problem, and with few exceptions initial anxiety or remoteness dissipated rapidly. All seemed to welcome the opportunity to speak of themselves at length, in privacy, and in detail to a nonjudgmental listener. All were given an opportunity at the end of the interview to ask the physician about matters of concern to them, and most thanked the interviewer for the opportunity to talk. Completing the recording form usually occupied an additional thirty minutes after the interview, and in order to avoid fatigue and to meet other requirements each person conducted only one interview on any given day. I held review sessions with both interviewers during my supervisory visits and also maintained regular contact with the clinic staff. Whenever possible I spoke informally with clients on the scene about their fertility-related experiences.

As cases accumulated on a nonselected basis, late users began to outnumber early users, so that the last several clients were selected on the basis of having had two or fewer children.

The 100 JFPA clients had come mainly for information, supplies, or scheduled followup visits. Just over one-fourth had experienced some undesirable effect from the current contraceptive and wanted to discuss the possibility of changing their method. Work with them was completed by late 1974.

To acquire a sample of 50 sexually active noncontracepting women, the interviewers spent several days in early 1975 acquainting themselves with the staff and setting of the Manley Clinic. The waiting room there was crowded in the mornings; patients had to wait approximately two hours before seeing the examining physician. When the interviewer arrived the chief nurse asked each patient of reproductive age (15-44), in order of arrival, whether or not she was using a contraceptive and whether she was sexually active. Patients invariably answered these questions directly. The first woman fitting the screening requirement was asked if she would be willing to talk with a physician as part of a research project, and was promised immediate attention for her or her child's medical complaint as a reward.

This group of nonusers did not differ from the JFPA group on the basis of the age of current children. Almost two-thirds came bringing their own children or those of neighbors, usually because of colds or diarrhea. None requiring care for themselves had a serious or incapacitating illness.

As at the JFPA clinic, acceptance of the invitation to talk was general, and the interview experience was similar, although the interviews were sometimes shorter because they involved no details of contraceptive use. Although they were not current users, 20 had used a contraceptive device or taken a pill at one time, but having discontinued did not plan to start again.

It had been initially planned to interview the mates of the women respondents, for a total of 150 men, with a subsample interviewed jointly in order to provide observations of couple interaction. A shorter data schedule for both the male and couple interviews was developed for this purpose. The interviewer was an experienced Jamaican male health worker, a longtime employee of JFPA. Past middle age, a man who elicited trust and confidence, he was selected over several applicants in a joint interview with me and the psychiatrist interviewers. After a period of training and observation he began his work. In two months of full-time effort, however, he was able to locate and interview only ten of the respondents' mates. In January 1974 I spent a full week with him, traveling about Kingston in search of male partners, observing his technique in the field, and reviewing his completed records. This experience significantly enriched my view of the city and gave me additional firsthand information about the working-class Kingston man's view of sex and reproduction. The sparse yield in respondents, however, in proportion to effort invested, led to a decision to abandon the original plan; instead, we decided to interview men coming to the JFPA clinic to obtain contraceptives (condoms) for themselves. The data recording schedule was revised accordingly for greater brevity and simplicity. Although it included some questions directly comparable with those for the women, many areas differed on the basis of gender role. The interviewer saw as many men as he could easily manage, on a consecutive arrival basis, five days weekly except for holidays until November 1, 1974. Each interview required from 30 minutes to one hour, and the schedule was further limited by the uneven presentation of clients. The heaviest period tended to be on Friday afternoons in preparation for what more than one client said he hoped would be "a busy weekend."

More men than women refused to be interviewed, perhaps because most were employed and had come expecting to pick up their condoms and depart in a relatively brief time. They were also more resistant to intrusion on their privacy, so that after the first week the interviewer discontinued requests for any identifying information such as name and address. Despite a refusal rate of approximately 20 percent, systematic data were collected on 283 male JFPA clients by the end of the allotted period.

Statistical Analysis

After coding and the compilation of initial frequency tables, the problem of statistical analysis was considered at length with professional consultants. The materials did not lend themselves to factor analysis or coefficients of correlation without the possibility of error, although it was considered that multiple regression analysis of specific items might be useful. Eventually we decided that simple percentages and gamma and gamma-type statistics would constitute the most useful and valid presentations. The latter permit a measure of relationship between two sets of ordered categories constructed from data involving uneven intervals (nonmonotonic series) between points. Gamma measures the predictability of order for one variable from the ordering of another (Meuller, Schuessler, and Costner, 1970). Thus, gamma gives an indication, for example, of the association of age of first coitus or conjugal union status or years of schooling, on one hand, with numbers of partners or type of contraceptive use or number of pregnancies or attitudes toward a grandmother on the other. For practical purposes the figure of .30 almost always indicates a probability of chance occurrence of from .05 to .001.

The trends revealed by statistical analysis, however, say little regarding the subjective experience, conflict resolution, or fertility-related decisions of a particular man or woman, singly or as a member of a couple. Information about group patterns depends upon measures that may obscure personally relevant issues. Moreover, the clean numbers emerging from a computer require careful viewing. They are at a considerable distance from and reflect significant transformations of the "dirty" data—the signs to which investigators respond and which they modify through their responses. That is why I am concerned not only with numbers, but, insofar as it is possible to record them, with respondent reports of direct experience, the immediate experience of interviewer and interviewee, my impressions of living in and with the society, and the comments of individuals to me and to my colleagues.

3   The Folk Context
of Sex and Reproduction

Some woman talk about tea, mamma look tea, mama look tea.
Some woman talk about tea, mamma look tea, mama look tea.
Come an drink de mazawatee ile a bush, an de tayma weed
But de young gal crazy fe de lignum vitae, oh mama look tea.
But de young gal crazy fe de lignum vitae, oh mama look tea.

De young gal talk about tea, mama look tea, mama look tea.
De young gal talk about tea, mama look tea, mama look tea.
Come an drink de mazawatee ile a bush, an de tayma weed
But de young gal crazy fe de lignum vitae, oh mama look tea.
But de young gal crazy fe de lignum vitae, oh mama look tea.

*Recorded in rural Jamaica and reproduced
with the permission of Olive Lewin*

Health and Fertility

The idea of doing something to keep one's body strong and healthy
is congenial to working-class Jamaicans. Most attempt to improve
themselves or even to treat real or fancied minor disorders before consulting a folk healer. Physicians, though respected, are
part of the authority structure; people are reluctant to confide
ideas that may subject them to ridicule or contempt: "Like me
from the country and not know about things." In this sense the
management of conditions and physiological rhythms is an accepted part of everyday life; it is not perceived as going against
nature, but rather as part of nature. Both tradition and the conditions of island life sustain comfort with and dependence upon
the natural in contrast to the technical world, despite awareness
of the curative powers of modern medicine.

"Tea" in particular is prominent in the Jamaican context of

health or bodily related behavior. It includes the range of non-alcoholic hot drinks, many of which would be regarded elsewhere as soups, broths, medicines, or specific preparations such as coffee or cocoa. It can refer simply to the morning meal, which for many poor people is in fact limited to an infusion of tea leaves or, in the country, some preferred local bark or leaf boiled in hot water to which sugar and sometimes lime are added.

The tea that is central in song or story is usually the medicinal infusion or magic potion made from "boiling a bush," local botanicals in the form of bark, twigs, roots, leaves, flowers, or weeds. *Ganja*, or marijuana, is known simply as "the herb" to its Rastafarian users, who may take it as tea as well as smoke it. It is used for colds, a range of minor physical ailments, asthmatic episodes, and sometimes menstrual discomfort. Ganja seed soaked in white rum for several months is known as a general tonic. Lignum vitae (*Guiacum officinale*), mentioned in the song above, yields a resin that is occasionally soaked in rum and used as a gargle for sore throat, a drink for "bellyache," and a salve for cuts and bruises. The juice of the leaves is sometimes taken in a tea for "biliousness." In earlier times the wood and bark were considered "good for" a variety of disturbances. The "hardest" wood in Jamaica, according to Lewin it has phallic significance in the song.

Few of the vegetable, animal, or mineral materials of everyday Jamaican life do not have some potential health-related use. Modern chemical products also form part of the island world view, designated by such concrete, familiar, and connotatively rich names as "horsehorn" for ammonia and "steel drops" for ferric chloride. Many of these substances are considered to have contraceptive, abortifacient, or potency- and fertility-inducing properties. Similarly, many "natural" practices, such as prolonging the lactation period, are recognized as means of delaying the next pregnancy. These suggest a strong interest in personal fertility regulation antedating the advent of technical methods, and—despite their ineffectiveness—their acceptability so long as they involve the familiar and natural.

The extent of actual current use of these methods for fertility regulation is unknown; information about personal attempts to keep from becoming pregnant or to stop pregnancy once initiated is often qualified by the statement that the informant herself does not do it but knows someone who does, or has simply heard of it. People especially "in the country" tend to be "quiet" about these matters; even friends do not talk much together about sex or "the control," and especially not about abortion, which is illegal. Nor are physicians customary recipients of information about indigenous or nonprescriptive methods of fertility regulation. Nurses in several settings were especially vehement about physician failure in this respect: patients say they are "afraid to tell the doctor anything like that . . . because he so high."

Two points of view prevail about birth control through nondrug methods, such as prolonged lactation, or with nonprescriptive chemicals and pharmaceuticals, including those intended for other purposes. One, voiced by the majority of informants, is that Jamaican women who do not use technical contraceptive methods simply have not made up their minds that their fertility should be limited. Those who have thought about it may occasionally use some "country" or folk approach in a half-hearted manner; but people who do this are not really convinced. A very few who are "Christian" (often Jehovah's Witnesses) use rhythm because they consider technical devices immoral. But once a woman has arrived at a decision she will go to a family planning clinic, a private physician, or a drugstore for technical information and supplies.

The other point of view, expressed forcefully by a number of nurses and other staff workers experienced in both clinical and informal country settings, is that a minority of women have decided to limit their fertility without using technical methods. Their avoidance may be due to a wish not to be seen at the family planning clinic; embarrassment at purchasing devices or pills from a drugstore; fear of the cancer- or bloodclot-inducing potential of the pill publicized in the popular press; fear that an IUD or condom may be lost somewhere in the body—"It will get up into your shoulder and you'll have to be operated"; or a vague concern that a method will make them "sick." These fears and concerns were all heard from one or another respondent in the systematic interviewing study. In general, as one nurse put it, most are "afraid of themselves . . . afraid to put a finger in their vagina," whether to retrieve a lost condom or to examine themselves.

This minority does not adhere permanently to the decision not to use technical methods. Sooner or later, despite their personal contraceptive efforts, additional pregnancies force women who wish to limit or space their children to overcome their fears and resistance and seek professional assistance. Since technical methods have become available, therefore, it appears that non-prescriptive approaches are used either by those not yet sure that they wish to regulate their own fertility or by those who would like to do so but resist technical methods until the cumulative hardship of additional unwanted pregnancies forces them, however reluctantly, to conclude that their own attempts are ineffective.

Finally, many women will not use a technical contraceptive because their mates accuse them of wishing to be promiscuous. Some will remove the IUD because their "man say it make it stink." Others have obtained contraceptives, but in hesitating to use them have wittingly or unwittingly allowed their mates to find them and throw them away. The differences between male and female attitudes toward contraception resemble those documented in earlier studies. Clarke (1957) observed mutual distrust between the sexes in rural areas in the 1940s and 1950s, with women inducing abortions with bush medicines and telling the disapproving men that they had fallen down and miscarried. Although most of Blake's (1961) female respondents approved of birth control most of the males did not, a prominent reason being fear of their mate's infidelity. Jamaica Family Planning Association "encouragement visitors" (1968-1969) reported that the most important reason given by women who had agreed to use contraceptives and did not do so was that their male partners had objected.

Botanical Substances

The most widely used folk medicines are made from the leaves, roots, and bark of plants that can be gathered in field or wood or grown in back yard or garden patch. These have been listed in detail by a number of investigators (Asprey and Thornton, 1953, 1955; Lowe, 1972; Campbell, 1974 a and b), but their effects in many instances remain uncertain. Some seem to be toxic; others are at best ineffective. None seems to have nutritive value. In general, the more astringent or sharper the taste, the greater the attributed power.

Preparation is most often by boiling in water to which other substances are added. The ensuing liquid may be reduced to an essence before being "strengthened" with wine or rum or other substances such as soot from wood fires. These "bush teas" or "bush medicines" are known to everyone in city and country alike, although their use by urban dwellers seems to be diminishing.

The mode of administration varies from internal consumption, especially for colds (a term designating almost any unexplained ache or pain), to external application in the form of soaks, lotions, baths, or oils for sprains or physical discomfort ranging from difficulty in breathing to painful menstruation. Bush baths may be very complex, requiring a great many specific ingredients. Some substances, used for "nerves," were often mentioned by psychiatric patients. The most frequently encountered was soursop (*Annona muricata*), whose leaf was used for an infusion both as a tonic and as a sedative. Like many Jamaican bush medicines, it has a history of use in other parts of the West Indies and in Africa. In Africa the whole plant reportedly is used for colds, coughs, and fever and the bark and root, which contain tannin, for dysentery and worms. In Grenada the leaves are used to make tea for fever ("to cool the blood"), colds, and coughs and as a sedative for vomiting (Asprey and Thornton, 1953). Like so many other bush medicines, its multiple applications suggest not only separate properties in leaf and bark but also a lack of specificity and the importance of context and expectation in its effect.

Almost all respondents in the study acknowledged at least a rare use of teas as a tonic or for medicinal purposes. None, however, admitted to using a botanical for fertility regulation, although the majority had "heard of" others doing so, and a few reported such use by relatives or personal friends. This indication of infrequent use coincides with the reports of staff members at various clinics. As one put it strongly, "Bush teas are out!" Another noted that in almost 15 years as a country midwife (in one of the more advanced parishes) she had not encountered a single instance in which bush medicines had been used for either contraception or abortion. She did feel, however, that there probably are some areas "dominated by a strong *nana* [an untrained midwife-herbalist] who grew up there and has been known to everyone all their lives," and that in these places botanicals may still be used. Despite these opinions, it is probable that a variety of plant substances are used occasionally for fertility control. Thus, a university clinic maid who often visited her family "in the country" said that although neither she nor her friends had ever done so she knew that in an emergency one could "boil a bush in the burn pan to keep from having baby."

The most frequently mentioned plant was pennyroyal, which according to various published accounts is boiled with cerasee, marigold, or a rusty nail for use as an abortifacient. Marigold itself was earlier reported (Beckwith, 1953) as a cure for menstrual troubles and, by implication, an abortifacient. Our informants rarely confronted the idea of pregnancy termination but tended instead to speak of "bringing down the period" when it had not "been seen" for a while. Similarly, the prescription for using marigold boiled with cerasee directed, "If menstruation ceases, drink as tea for nine mornings."

The reported medical uses of pennyroyal include treatment for diarrhea and stomachache (Campbell, 1974b) and a "rather curious 'cure' for a catarrhal cold in which a poultice of beaten leaves moistened with rum is applied to a small bare patch on top of the head" (Asprey and Thornton, 1953). "The water will run out of your nose and cure the complaint" (Beckwith, 1927). Our informants were unfamiliar with the cure for catarrh but knew about its presumed laxative properties: "Take it for a washout."

Men as well as women had heard of the fertility regulating use of "pennyriall," said by several to be part of the regular garden of nanas "in the hills." Four or five stalks of this are boiled with cobweb from the blackening on the kitchen shed ceiling made by putting green grass on the fire. The liquid, reduced from about one and a half quarts to a pint, is drunk by the wineglass, perhaps with a bit of wine or nutmeg added, for the nine mornings. This is said to "bring back" the missed period. Other informants included a clinic maid: "Take it if you don't see your period a month . . . Country people know about it." A young Kingston-born stenographer: "I heard in school, if you miss your period, boil it and drink it." A nurse: "Nanas use it for postdelivery hemorrhage and also for abortions. Most have it growing in their yards." An old man, a caretaker at a general medical clinic: "It was used a long time ago in the country at St. Mary . . . I never saw it in town, don't know if it works . . . but they come looking for the weed, a young man and a girl." A St. Andrew housewife: ". . . can still get it in the market . . . I never see it used, but hear of it." A domestic worker from St. Andrew: "It was used in the old days, but not since 'the planning' came in." A 35-year-old domestic just returned from working in Philadelphia: "My auntie had it in her yard . . . I think it more used in Kingston than we know."

These comments suggest that pennyroyal has a secure place in the indigenous armamentarium. On the other hand, doubt is cast on its general occurrence and use by the fact that one former country midwife was totally unfamiliar with it.

Cerasee is listed in all available reference works as an abortifacient and in Grenada (Asprey and Thornton, 1953) was reportedly taken monthly as a contraceptive. It was not, however, so identified by any of our informants, the majority of whom were familiar with it only as a common medicinal tea and tonic. A college student, for example, said her grandmother had recommended it to her for "pain in the tummy." A barmaid had used it "for bellyache." Others noted its use "to purify the blood" or "to rub on to cool skin with a fever."

The fruity pulp of calabash has been used to "force the menses" and to "clean out the womb" after childbirth (Asprey and Thornton, 1953). A midwife and a nurse had heard that "when nanas deliver a baby they mix it (calabash) inside with castor oil." This pulp is given to the postpartum woman for nine days to facilitate expulsion of "retained products." These do not refer to placental remnants, but to the undefined cause of occasional postpartum lassitude or depression.

Ram-goat dashalong (*Turnera ulmifolia*) leaves boiled as tea make a frequent beverage and cold remedy, used also for prickly heat, constipation, and weakness. Although various published sources report it as an abortifacient, only one respondent, a nurse who travels between rural clinics, knew of this use. As she said, it has been used to "attempt abortion, but less and less, because now you can get an abortion on the side so the younger people coming up don't know too much about it." This nurse was also the only informant who had heard of the possible use of bamboo leaf by "some country people who boil it for tea to try to produce abortion."

Thyme boiled as a tea may produce a "purge or washout." Although it is not mentioned in the literature for this purpose, a number of informants cited it as a frequently tried but ineffective abortifacient. One person said her grandmother had used it to help remove her afterbirth. A middle-class JFPA worker said she had heard of its use to induce "painless labor." The old man previously mentioned said, "When you have a baby, boil, take a cup if having labor pain and can't get through." A domestic had heard of its use "when hard to give birth," and one of the clinic nurses said that she thought it was sometimes used to stop postpartum bleeding.

None of the many other botanicals described in the literature as contraceptives or abortifacients elicited any sign of recognition from the informants. The substances named above, however, and the nature of the comments about them indicate the continuing prominence of these folk medicines in the Jamaicans' perception of the world around them and in their perceived ability to regulate their own bodily processes.

Chemicals and Other Substances

Like people elsewhere, Jamaicans use materials at hand, including those designated for other purposes, to attempt control of their fertility when strongly enough impelled to do so. As one physician put it, women who don't want to be pregnant but are not sufficiently motivated to seek technical help depend on "teas, washouts, and purges," especially castor oil and douches. Perhaps most common is a douche of warm water with a little vinegar or soap, used to wash out the sperm immediately after intercourse. Red Stripe beer, the only kind originating on the island, is used precoitally as a contraceptive and postcoitally as a douche. Royal Blue, designed for laundry purposes, is used as a douche in warm water before or after intercourse, or is taken orally with water or stout as a contraceptive or abortifacient. "Taking the Blue" is also common among prostitutes before a ship is due "in order to prevent the period." Similarly, drinking a mixture of vinegar and water just after menstruating was reported by an old woman at the Manley Clinic as a country method to avoid conceiving during the next month. Quinine tablets are inserted intravaginally as a contraceptive or taken by mouth with white rum in an effort to produce abortion.

Perhaps the most widely used though almost always ineffective abortifacient is castor oil taken orally. Drinking hot gin and stout together was also reported from the West Kingston slum, along with "purges and washouts" to attempt abortion.

Other Methods of Fertility Control

All informants agreed that prolonged lactation is the most frequent means of attempting fertility control on the island. They could not agree, however, whether women depending on this method have seriously decided to limit their fertility. Lactation is rarely used for more than two years as a means of contraception. Pregnant women not infrequently note that they are surprised to have a "new baby come" when they are still nursing their last.

Abstinence for younger people with no or few children was reported to be significant only if the woman "did not have a boy friend." One informant, for example, volunteered that she had not had a male friend, and therefore no coitus, for two years after her husband's death and for this reason was not at risk of pregnancy. A few couples apparently limit frequency of intercourse without particular reference to the ovulatory cycle simply on the supposition that the fewer the ejaculations the smaller the chance of conception. The only couples for whom abstinence is apparently an accepted means of avoiding pregnancy are those who already have several (variously defined as four to six) children. In these instances many informants noted, and staff members in group discussions generally agreed, that the woman might delay resumption of coitus for as long as a year after delivery. Kingston informants and younger couples conceded that the man probably has sexual relations with other women during this time. In the country, however, and among older couples, the male partners are regarded as more cooperative and do not engage in intercourse with other women because they are "dedicated."

Coitus interruptus was reported by few of the respondents in the clinic study. All other informants regarded this method as rare. Some volunteered that Jamaican men would not withdraw, feeling that it would be bad for them to do so. Male family planning clients did not regard this as an acceptable or effective method, and some said this was why they came regularly for condoms. A few stated that they could not and did not want to engage in the kind of self-control that this required.

One general practitioner reported that a few of his male medical patients told him they practiced anal intercourse with their mates in order to avoid pregnancy. Respondents were not asked about this specific method and none volunteered using it. No other physician or nurse reported such information upon questioning, and none had encountered a woman complaining of rectal tears or other difficulties suggesting regular anal intercourse.

Fertility and Potency

In the course of regular interviews some informants commented on the use of bush medicines to increase fertility or potency. Both client and staff respondents agreed that occasionally women unable to conceive consult Obeahmen, who give them "something to drink." This is true in urban Kingston as well as in rural areas.

Several informants said that in the country some people drink a tea made of sempervivum or Sinkle-Bible (*Aloe vera*) to "put it back," that is, to restore semen in men and sexual energy in both sexes. In the past this has been reported as a means of promoting menstrual flow. A tea made of the boiled leaf and an essence made from steeping the leaf in white rum are well-known remedies for colds and indigestion. One young man volunteered that in his personal experience teas made of coconut root and the inner core of bamboo were especially good to "put it back." The chief of the Manley Clinic reported being consulted by a number of men concerned with their potency. These were chiefly in their fifties and sixties who, because their mates were younger, were still, she said, "on the sexual treadmill." At all ages, according to many physicians and nurses, Jamaican men consume vast quantities of malt (one well-known brand being advertised as "the big drink"), stout (one brand is advertised to "put it back"), and other products with enhancement or restoration of potency as the conscious aim.

Several male and a number of female informants noted that women may judge men on the basis of sexual performance and make fun of them if they are not competent. Even educated women have been heard to comment that they "can go on longer sexually," that is, to a later age, than men.

Male attitudes toward fellatio and cunnilingus suggest a latent perception of women as fundamentally dangerous. Interviews with male psychiatric patients and informal conversations with colleagues, social acquaintances, and workers such as clinic janitors revealed no special feeling about fellatio other than an occasionally expressed wish that they could have it more often. Lower-class men, however, were almost unanimous in their feelings that cunnilingus was unmasculine or deviant, put one "in the woman's power," or exposed one to dangerous, possibly poisonous substances—a point of view embodied in at least one recorded song. As one man stated, "Eating pussy like eating poison."

Surgical Abortion

During the study period, abortion was illegal on the island except to save the life of the mother. The evidence was overwhelming, however, that it was practiced and often under unfavorable circumstances. Estimates of illegally performed procedures range up to 25,000 yearly, but there is no exact information about the prevalence or incidence of abortion. Several cases of septic after-effects were identified during this time. Informants said that most abortions are performed by pharmacists passing catheters through the cervix into the uterus. One informant had used a knitting needle. None knew of the cervical insertion of sticks or twigs such as the "slippery elm" used in the rural United States. Well-to-do women go to Miami, England, or Canada or are sometimes able to have their own gynecologists perform abortions in Jamaica.

Of the 150 JFPA clients and Manley Clinic patients interviewed, 133 had been pregnant at least once. Among these, the rate of stillbirths and induced and spontaneous abortions ranged from 3.8 percent for those with one pregnancy to 22.7 percent for those with six. The high positive correlation between the number of live births and total unsuccessful pregnancies (gamma .68) may reflect the increasing use of abortion among multiparous women as a desperate attempt never to have more babies, or it may reflect—as suggested by the high proportion reported as stillborn—increasing physical impairment. Many women express strong negative feelings about having more babies without the personal or socioeconomic support of marriage. Thus, perinatal neglect of self and newborn infant or failure to obtain adequate prenatal care may reflect an unconscious attempt to abort. In this sense a stillbirth or neonatal death may be regarded as a self-induced extrauterine abortion.

All respondents knew about consciously sought abortion, but their expressed attitudes to using it themselves varied widely. Few were unequivocally in favor of its use on demand. Many more, however, agreed that under certain circumstances—including those when a child was unwanted for economic or social reasons—it should be available. But most, especially those with only one or two children, were concerned with its possible dangers. Fears of dying, becoming sick, and becoming sterile were all mentioned. As one put it, "I thought about it, but too dangerous. Life in jeopardy and all that." Several felt that everything should be weighed. A traditional ("no clapping") Baptist said, "It hard to make up your mind, but sometimes you have to decide even if don't tell anyone and stay quiet about it." Some mentioned its sinful connotations, but only in reference to themselves. Despite personal reservations, they felt that others should be free to seek it if they wished. Only one, a Catholic, specifically stated, "It not right to kill." Most of those who did mention moral values did not claim this as their central reason but referred to the value of children, especially the first child. One woman said, "My religion also say you should be chaste till you marry, and I don't. When I first didn't see my period and was upset I thought of losing it. But I decided to keep the child because I knew I would love it, and maybe would never have more."

African Influences on Folk Culture

Possible African contributions to Jamaican attitudes toward fertility remain a matter of conjecture. Approximately 91 percent of the population is officially designated as African or Afro-European and another approximately 5 percent as of mixed African, East Indian, Oriental, or other descent; only 0.8 percent is classed as European (JIS, 1970). Sensitive observers like Lewin (1973) consider the African world view fundamental to the unexplicated attitudes of the uneducated, still rurally rooted, majority of Jamaicans, for whom an elemental and creative life force makes reproduction a fundamentally valued behavior, while contraception and abortion are antithetical and for some abhorrent. They keep their traditions alive through a host of unwritten and unchoreographed songs and dances, many of which are appropriate to birth, puberty, and marriage, although most are associated with death, perhaps a consequence of the short life span and the prominence of separation in the consciousness of the slave. (St. Thomas Parish records from 1831 showed the average life span for a Negro slave born in Jamaica to be 26 years [Norris, 1962].)

The major cult of possible fertility-related significance is Kumina, which flourishes mainly in the remote, backward areas of the countryside and in the slum areas of Kingston. It is reputed to remain strong in the parish of St. Thomas, the highest fertility area adjacent to the metropolis. Kumina practice varies but usually includes drumming, dancing, spirit possession, and occasional animal sacrifice. Kumina cult groups are frequently led by a "Queen . . . usually a middle-aged woman of a very arresting personality"; this type of female leader may exemplify "the quite commonly held belief among African peoples of the woman as the life giving force and symbol of the great earth mother," a belief that some consider fundamental to traditional Jamaican resistance to birth control (Lewin, 1973, p. 6).

In the revival movements noted in chapter 5, spirit healing and ritual baths may have fertility-related significance; among other problems, they deal with sterility, impotence, venereal disease, apparent pregnancy extending beyond the time of expected delivery, and gaining the affection of or taking revenge upon a lover. Informal conversation suggests that although abortion may sometimes be desired, it is not usually identified in unequivocal terms and may not even be clearly conceptualized by the subject, who identifies the problem as one of missing menses rather than one of unexpected pregnancy; the subject seeks to "bring down" a "period which does not come."

Balm yards exist in both rural and urban places throughout the island. Here the sick consult their "shepherds" for help. These are charismatic, respected healers and religious leaders sometimes feared (as in the earlier Native Baptist variety), and often venerated by members of their flock, who act as staff members and supporters. The belief systems that support them, though never tabulated and only reluctantly acknowledged to outsiders, appear to be widespread.

The healing in balm yards is both herbal and ritual in the pattern of people who believe that sickness, like other human difficulty, is fundamentally caused by spiritual forces. The healing is directed both to bodily disease and to emotional and social problems, including the stimulation, prevention, and sometimes, reputedly, termination of pregnancy.

Disturbances for which people seek assistance are sometimes

The Rastafarian movement and the rise of African nationalism have permitted Africa to influence contemporary Jamaican life by serving as a symbol for a people in search of an identity. For years anything African was denigrated, and West Indians seemed to find their models, however ambivalently, in the customs, values, and physical appearance of the people who had colonized them. After emancipation, British whites constituted a major emulative reference group, historically expressed in the saying "Every John Crow think him pickney white, and every jackass think him cubby racehorse pickney" (Jekyll, 1904). This emulation was apparent in the importance attributed to correct formal dress, including ties and dark suits in the hottest weather, until the bush-jacket vogue initiated by Prime Minister Michael Manley in 1974. It remains in the exaggeratedly English names given to children, the interest in cricket, the social value of British schooling among the upper classes, the prominent place accorded members of the Royal Family in the local media, the continuing prestige of Anglican Church attendance, and conversations of the well-to-do sprinkled with references to BOAC and one's London flat.

Even in recent years, tests of self-concept given to Jamaican adolescents revealed the ideal body type to be Caucasian, with dissatisfaction about one's appearance increasing with dark skin color, "bad" hair, and broad nose and lips (Phillips, 1973). These responses, however, emerged in the context of a new but still uncertain pride in blackness; changing values are leading to new self-concepts related, among other factors, to the ideas of negritude and black power (Nettleford, 1970).

The new symbolic strength of Africa has been dramatically reflected in its appeal for the poorest Jamaicans: "In the dense slum areas the prevailing doctrine is now Rastafari" (Smith, Augier, and Nettleford, 1960). The accelerating acceptance of the Rastafari among the middle class and the adoption by politically conscious Jamaican university students of some aspects of Rastafarian dress, hairstyle, behavior, and belief all reflect a new pride and activism in African identity as opposed to that of former slave and colonial pawn. All these developments follow historically from Marcus Garvey's early and for a time forgotten "glory in the fact that he was a full-blooded black man without any taint of white blood in his veins" (Cronon, 1969, p. 5).

The religion of the Rastafari, fundamentally Old Testament in nature, is oriented to Ethiopia and the divinity of Haile Selassie. The biblical books of Numbers and of Leviticus are quoted as forbidding the trimming of hair. Long matted hair is proof of the connection with Jah, the living god. Along with the beard, these "dreadlocks" represent the mane of the lion, a symbol of Ethiopia, and the beard and locks of Selassie himself. Rastafarianism has no similarities to the Afro-Jamaican cults, despised as reflecting white influence and submissiveness to extranatural spirits. The Rastas regard black people as the true Israelites. Beyond Jah Ras Tafari, the Creator, resides in every man. The Rasta, one with Jah, therefore refers to himself as "I *and* I." Man is God.

Although they are still a small minority of Jamaicans, the increasing visibility and acceptance of the Rastafari are important aspects of the context of fertility behavior, for they offer an identity opposed to the values promulgated by the government, JFPA, and other local groups collaborating with international agencies. A Jamaican scholar recently summarized the degree to which the movement symbolizes rejection of a total socioculture embodying white values with colonial roots: "The basis . . . was the racial and cultural suppression of poor blacks in a colonial environment where religion, music, art, education, self-respect, dignity, power and influence all derived from and reflected European attributes, character and control, and a denial of the worth of Afro-Jamaicans" (Stone, 1973, p. 154).

I regularly encountered Rastafari ideas in conversation with clinic and hospital patients and to a lesser degree with family planning clients. These ideas were also prominent in the popular press. On the few occasions when I examined Rastafarians themselves, mainly in the Casualty Department after they had been beaten by police (as possible ganja sellers), I inquired about their fertility-related beliefs. All male, they stressed the importance of continued fertility, distrust of any government-sponsored attempt to limit birth rates, and religious opposition to any attempt to interfere with the natural processes of their women, called "queens." Sex with one's queen during her menses is forbidden by biblical injunction. Abortion, tubal ligation, and chemical or mechanical contraception they call "internal murder." The movement itself is an essentially masculine phenomenon requiring utter female conformity. The woman stays faithful to her man, covers her head at all times, and never tries to straighten her hair. It is the black man much more than the woman who has called for continuing high levels of fertility and at times labeled contraceptive campaigns as white-sponsored programs of "genocide."

Recent studies have demonstrated that within Jamaica positive attitudes toward black power and the Rastafari are inversely related to occupational class and, by implication, lighter skin color (Stone, 1973). Much of the remaining significance of dark color is expressed in behavior related to economic status: "the frequent denigration of persons in subordinate roles . . . the high sensitivity of the manual classes to acts and statements that suggest . . . status denigration [and] the class biased nature of the treatment meted out to persons of lowly status by most persons in authority (irrespective of their class position)" (Stone, 1973, p. 120). Few women and no men in our clinic populations, however, made unequivocally negative statements about close relationships with whites. More than half the women stated that the heroine in a story about which comment was invited would accept a white man's proposal to keep her in return for sexual intercourse. Women with more children by more men tended to indicate that they themselves would respond positively to any offer of help. But very few men responded similarly: more than one-third said the heroine would reject the proposal outright, and about half stated that her decision would depend upon her personal circumstances.

Shared Categories and Their Private Meanings

The folk and medical approaches to sex, fertility, and reproduction involve several fundamental, overlapping ideas.

    1. The materials used are natural or nonnatural. One or one's

friends or relatives can grow, find, or gather natural substances without recourse to specially trained strangers. Natural procedures are already known to older members of the community, particularly women. Their use does not entail the risk of harmful consequences or loss of control, such as getting lost in the body. Manufactured items or chemicals, in contrast, must be obtained from a drugstore or clinic; they require the participation of people alien to the community; and they may have harmful consequences, such as impaired fertility or reduced potency, sexual desire, or "nature"; or they may elude control by the user. For some these nonnatural items represent an unexplicated spiritual threat by their lack of congruity with the high value attached to producing and sustaining life. For a few that threat is explicit: the use of a nonnatural contraceptive conflicts with specific religious beliefs. Nonnatural items differ from those that are part of the regular experience of everyday life since childhood.

2. Fertility-influencing materials or acts are strong or weak and certain processes are strengthening or weakening. Botanicals with intense tastes or odors may be physiologically powerful, producing good effects. Metal devices may also be powerful, but are dangerous: an IUD, for example, can "suck you down." Sexual relations are thought by some to be essential to mental health, but many believe them to have an essentially weakening effect on the body. Malt, stout, and other drinks are strong and able to restore sexual vigor after intercourse. The sexual urge reflects the presence of a person's "nature," and—predictably—acting upon that urge weakens or lessens that nature. Menstrual flow, however, is not weakening and its regular appearance is a sign of health; the discharge of unnecessary blood has a strengthening effect. Having children represents social strength. It also represents a kind of sexual-natural strength, reflecting a strong nature, potency, ability to have intercourse and "put it back," and highly valued procreative capacity. A person with no children is socially weak and may also be viewed as naturally weak.

3. The interior of the body is a mysterious place in which devices can become lost. The various apertures—vagina, urethra, anus, mouth, ears—all interconnect inside. Certain parts of the

interior may suck up or attract devices. Similarly, energy or strength residual in the interior may be sucked out, discharged, or otherwise depleted. Or the interior may react in an unpredictably unfavorable way to putting things in it: an IUD, for example, may "make it stink." It is undesirable to put foreign objects into body apertures. Even putting one's finger into the vagina may entail an unspecified risk. Yet the interior is the place in which babies grow and from which in time they are expelled.

4. Certain acts are magico-religious, whereas others with related aims are medical. Specialists qualified by personality as well as by training and experience carry out each category or act. Magico-religious acts, which are more familiar and employ natural substances, are usually preferred in initial efforts to deal with illness or discomfort, sometimes involving sexual-reproductive functions. These acts are less apt than medical ones to conflict with spiritual values.

5. Certain substances, items, or acts have shared symbolic value; that is, they are perceived by almost everyone as having a complex of meanings other than what they directly signify. The marigold, for example, may represent beauty, growth, springtime, or an unwanted pregnancy. A man's simultaneous maintenance of three sexual partners or his accumulation of children may directly reflect his sexual-affiliative urges. But because children are public manifestations of potency and power, these acts also symbolize his need to build a social support system and his striving for masculine status.

I take it for granted that all public symbols and shared action patterns have private meanings. A marigold in the hands of a menopausal woman may symbolize her wish to be a child in her mother's garden again; when she takes it to the hospital it may simply represent a connection with her home, where she and not the medical staff is in control of her body.

A man complaining of stomach discomfort reported a dream of a lion. He said it represented Haile Selassie, the Lion of Judah, and he spoke ecstatically of his wish to be part of the court of the divine emperor. But his associations led from a fat lion to a pregnant animal and thence to the fact that his woman was pregnant. From here his rambling conversation led to two divergent but related lines of fantasy. One was his wish to have his woman care for him like a baby. The other concerned his observations of her expanding belly, which interfered with his appetite for food, and his development of morning nausea. The public symbol of the potent lion had private meanings that were unfathomable through common sense or ordinary social participant-observation. The socially shared wish to have children as an expression of masculine power coexisted here with unconscious wishes both to produce children as an identification with powerful women and to be the child oneself, retaining the woman as a protecting mother and not having to compete for nurturance with her other children.

4   The Place: Kingston, Metropolis of a Rural Island

> . . . this land of bondage . . . this land of Babylon which de white slave masters call Jamaica.
>
> *A Rastafarian, in H.O. Patterson,* The Children of Sisyphus
>
> Doan' like de pressure here, an' me head botherin' me for money . . . Would like to take my chile' an' move back to the country . . . but now have no place to go.
>
> *Ethel A.*

The island is the physical entity in which Jamaicans live, work, love, have sexual intercourse, reproduce, and rear their children. What meanings does this context symbolize and reinforce in the lives of specific individuals? The nature of the place in which behavior occurs and the cultural forms that exist there can facilitate personal gratification of inadmissible needs without generating conscious conflict; by hindering gratification, it may stimulate development of alternative expressive, symbolic, or need-gratifying behaviors.

The Context of Experience and Behavior

The subjective reality of Kingston for our informants is suggested by the views of Ethel A., the 26-year-old mother of three children by two men. Her precarious livelihood depends partly on their occasional contributions to the support of the children she has had "for them," and on money from a current boy friend who would like her to "have a baby for" him. She and the children she already has, ages two, three, and five, live in a ramshackle building without piped water in the West Kingston slum, where she arrived from the country seeking work when she was 18. She leaves them with a friend when she goes out on occasional house-cleaning jobs. Another child, age seven, is with its father's mother in St. Thomas. Aware of her uncertain future, fearful that her single room will be robbed, she would like to move away; but she feels "stuck" in her tenement yard. Her grandmother has died, her mother is "in America," and her father—whom she has not seen for years—has his own woman. With no place to go, ready to succumb to "the pressure," she feels trapped, angry, and despairing in what she calls "Babylon."

When I first encountered Ethel in the hospital outpatient clinic where she had come seeking "medicine" for a headache, her reference to Babylon startled me. At first I thought she might be suffering from a delusion of persecution. Then, realizing she was indeed economically trapped and seemingly exploited by men who used her as a reproductive mechanism, I thought Babylon might stand for a chaotic, stressful sexual environment. Eventually I learned from her and others that this view emanated from the small but highly visible cult of the Rastafarians, who, feeling themselves African (now a symbol of anticolonialism), regard Jamaica as an oppressed and oppressing society dominated at long range by white Europeans and their lackeys, "the Babylon which holds them in the captivity of a protracted diaspora" (Nettleford, 1970, p. 41). Babylon is a major theme in Rex Nettleford's *Mirror, Mirror*; for him it is a code word for a society dominated by the economic imperialists of the North Atlantic countries, including the United States. For the Rastafarians it is a reason not to engage in gainful employment, since such work contributes to the support of a society they regard as corrupt. For me the concept was epitomized in the discontinuities of the city of Kingston: a sense of incoherence embodied in its jumble of palatial residences, tenements and shanties; its foreign businesses in the new high-rise buildings on streets filled with ragged sidewalk vendors; its smoke-belching trucks jostling for road space with handcarts; and its white visiting dignitaries come to consult with "brown man government" (Nettleford, 1970) in a sea of black faces. These disparities, of course, are no more fundamental than those found in most human civilizations. And Kingston does have a particular advantage. "The country," though poor and stingy, remains a green, familiar haven for those who can return to it. Ethel and others like her, however, often find it difficult to do so. At first she gave the most apparent reasons for not going back: she would have no work, no place to live, and no source of support. But then she spoke of the woman with whom her father now lives. "She hate me . . . maybe put spell on me, because me no want her." Babylon, in addition to its shared cultural and political influences, has for her a private, personal symbolism—oppression by the world of men, fathers, and sexual partners whom she simultaneously needs and distrusts. It means loneliness and lack of intimacy amidst multitudes. "The country" as an ideal is less the green rural haven of banana trees, poinsettia, and freedom from the fear of assault than it is the remembered place of childhood nurturance by a trusted, loving mother and grandmother. Recollection, however, is difficult in the dull surroundings of the clinic; after a few minutes she reminds me that she did come, after all, for medicine. Like poor Baltimoreans and the Cariocas of Rio de Janeiro, she yearns for a substance that can be swallowed or for an injection, some concrete aid for personal misery. In this situation I behave as the other doctors do. Unable to offer our patients love, care, and opportunity for mutual trust, we give them a chemical substance instead. The drug satisfies their immediate need; it also keeps us safely at a distance from each other.

An Island Identity

Even in the thick tension and sweaty heat of inner-city Kingston its inhabitants understand Jamaica as a Caribbean entity. People of all social classes speak familiarly of relatives and friends on other islands. They occasionally express feelings of rivalry or contempt—Jamaicans for Trinidadians, people of African descent for those of East Indian descent—but there is also a sense of community, especially about the nations that still feel themselves part of the British Commonwealth. Awareness of living on a small island is constant, and I quickly began to share this perception. The land base, approximately 146 by 51 miles, its blue water boundaries rarely out of sight, permits few illusions about expansive career possibilities and makes it easy to contemplate emigration as a solution to socioeconomic and personal problems.

As part of the former British West Indies, despite independence in 1962 the country retains close social, cultural, and political ties with Britain. The Jamaican Civil Service still offers paid "home leave" to Britain every three years for civil servants of a certain rank. Nearby Cuba, 90 miles north, is politically significant for leaders who view their nation as part of the Third World and as a separate political and economic identity from the United States.

Yet the island is indubitably within the geographic and communicative sphere of North America. Miami, described by some modestly affluent Jamaicans as "the great shopping center," is just over an hour's flying time from Kingston. Announcers who read the weather forecasts for the Jamaica Broadcasting Corporation describe weather conditions on the eastern seaboard of the United States in great detail, not only because cold waves sweeping across the continent influence the weather and the tourist industry, but also because wealthy Jamaicans make frequent trips there and want to know the temperatures they are likely to encounter. Real and imagined political and social influences on the island, sometimes from Canada but especially from the United States, are subject to occasional distortion and magnification. Although the United States is not widely identified with the population program, it has been accused of genocidal intentions against not only Jamaicans but black people in general.

At the same time, the United States is recognized by many as the source of good things, spiritual as well as material. American evangelists in the Caribbean are welcomed with fervor. Poor Jamaicans may make regular donations to Oral Roberts and others whose sermons and requests reach them by radio. Many go back and forth to the United States, working intermittently as domestics or day laborers. Ethel A. finds it easier to think of finding a job in Baltimore, Philadelphia, or New York than in the parish of St. Thomas where she was born, a short bus trip from Kingston.

The Land

Outside Kingston the coastal plains, which support a number of fishing villages, are largely devoted to agriculture. The interior, however, is so rugged and mountainous that only 20 percent of the total land area has been classified as arable. These mountains with their overhanging rain clouds are partly responsible for the richness of the cultivated soil. An estimated 38 percent of the adult labor force is directly engaged in farming, and more than half the population depends largely upon the soil for a livelihood (Floyd, 1970).

Country dwellers on the steeper hills and mountains grow subsistence crops on small, often eroded lots rarely exceeding five acres. Bananas, plantains, yams, sweet potatoes, and breadfruit provide the basis for their predominantly starchy diet. There are some legumes, citrus—mostly limes—and a great variety of other fruits. Mangoes are especially prized; bakers sell less bread at mango time. The country people supplement their diet when they can by raising a cow, a few chickens, a goat, or a pig or two.

On the level areas the major crop is sugar grown on large, mechanized plantations. The dark-skinned, weatherbeaten cane cutter, a sweaty rag tied about his forehead and a machete in his hand, is a familiar sight in the narrow lanes surrounding the fields. Bananas, rum, coffee, spices, citrus, and tobacco also have significant economic value. So, too, has ganja; although the marijuana trade is illegal, it is possibly the country's major cash crop and is widely blamed as the economic basis for the import of guns to the island. A few large landholders who raise fodder on the more gentle slopes and rolling hills breed dairy and beef cattle.

The other Jamaican product of major economic significance is bauxite. The large processing plants provide employment for many and are like self-contained states, offering their workers health and social services as well as salaries out of scale with those available elsewhere in the local economy. To be one of the "bauxite boys" is an enviable status for a Jamaican worker, and exuberantly driven bauxite trucks are among the hazards of the narrow mountain highways.

Population Distribution

The least populated areas are high and rugged. Pleasant land and water and the early incidence of disease determined the sites of military posts, farming settlements, market centers, and resorts. Newcastle, a military camp of the original British occupation troops and of today's Jamaica Defense Force, moved from the plain to the mountains above Kingston to escape the unhealthy miasma of the coastal swamps.

Jamaica is divided into thirteen parishes with population centers of varying size and complexity. Most country towns have populations of 2,000 to 6,000, but rural areas such as those around May Pen and Mandeville are densely inhabited. The places identified as urban in the 1970 census, accounting for 41.4 percent of the population, were centers of 2,500 or more that possessed facilities indicating "some degree of modern living" such as banks, electricity, schools, libraries, and cinemas. Also taken into account were "the location of markets, shops, post offices, churches, court houses, tax offices, police stations and health facilities . . . whether or not roadways were paved [and] whether or not there was a piped water supply" (Bulletin 1, 1973, p. 14). The presence or lack of these features defines the context of early experience: carrying water from the standpipe, sometimes a center of social exchange, is part of daily life for large numbers of Jamaicans identifying themselves as either country or city people. There are few of the former without extensive adult experience in urban areas, and almost none of the latter who do not maintain close connections with relatives "in the country." Country relatives seem especially important for women living alone with their children in Kingston as they maintain a real or fancied feeling of intimacy with someone else.

The areas of highest fertility tend to be in the more remote, rugged uplands, comparatively isolated from modern values and attitudes. The ratio of children aged 0-4 years to women aged 15-44 years in these regions is 90-94 percent, compared with 55-59 percent in urban areas, with small towns and lowland plantation areas in between (Eyre, 1972a, p. 39). Population size in the highlands, however, remains low because of outmigration. Conversely, lowlands characterized by high fertility and high rates of natural increase show a higher proportion of people of reproductive age as a consequence of inmigration.

St. Ann's Parish, site of the oldest and most consistently offered family planning service on the island, has the lowest birthrate. A local physician suggested that this may be partly the result of a great number of tubal ligations performed at a clinic there during the 1960s. St. Thomas, with the lowest rate of contraceptive acceptors per 1,000 females, 38.5 in 1970-71, is one of the least industrialized and, despite its proximity to Kingston, least literate parishes. According to 1970 data, it had the largest number of births per mother (4.07) and per parish woman (3.56), and of mothers with more than three children (60.2 percent). Here, absence of opportunities for self-determination through employment and education coexists with failure to use available family planning information and services.

The major population center after Kingston is Montego Bay, with 43,754 inhabitants. A place of hotel and restaurant enclaves walled off from the roads and filled with white U.S. and Canadian tourists, Jamaicans call it the "Republic of Mo' Bay" and perceive it as an entity separate from the rest of the country. The next most populous area, Spanish Town, the former national capital and now parish capital of St. Catherine, with 40,731 inhabitants, is immediately contiguous to the Kingston Metropolitan Area.

The Kingston Metropolitan Area

Kingston is situated on the south side of the island, separated from the major tourist areas by a mountain range in the parish of St. Andrew. The Kingston-St. Andrew Corporate Area, also known as the Kingston Metropolitan Area, or KMA, included 850,000 people, almost half the official national total of 1,865,400, at the time of the 1970 census. It contains 63.3 percent of the island's urban and approximately 40 percent of its total population. It is estimated that despite increasing outmigration, especially of middle- and upper-income people since 1975, at least 6,000 new household units are formed there annually (Eyre, 1979). Montego Bay, Spanish Town, May Pen, and Mandeville account for another 20 percent of the urban dwellers. A large population, however, does not necessarily mean a modern world view or a collective sense of self similar to that of the urban proletariat of industrialized nations. Jamaican city and town dwellers, struggling with odd jobs for individual survival, often continue to perceive themselves as rooted in the country and seem to lack a common investment in the status of salaried industrial workers.

From Country to City and Back

Country people from other parishes, impelled by poverty, monotony, lack of land for personal exploitation, lack of educational facilities for children, and lack of a personal future, come to Kingston fully understanding that they will be underemployed. Nevertheless some still seek excitement and imagine that city life will offer something to replace the old emptiness. Many of the young people, in their teens and early twenties, with whom I talked at the hospital, at the health or family planning centers, or in shopping centers or fast-food shops, spoke of "escape." "Me decide to get away" was a frequent theme. "Getting away" meant avoiding the discipline of parents, or especially grandparents, and the tiring routine of work in the fields or household chores. Others, mainly teenagers and young adults, came looking vaguely for work, excitement, anything but living their lives as cane cutters or in villages or on mountain slopes. Many who, like Ethel A., wished to return to the country after a few years, had come, despite their knowledge of Kingston's dismal prospects, looking for jobs that could give them the money they imagined would grant independence.

Anxiety about crime causes a constant stream of migrants to make their way back to the country in search of security for themselves and their families. A 1973 survey of central Kingston showed that despite friendship ties and low rents, many householders considered leaving because of "gangs and violence" (Norton, 1978, p. 70). Gentle's earlier survey (1968) reported that 41.5 percent of householders in Jonestown were considering moving away from the area. Some sample surveys have shown that "the actual rate of movement in Western Kingston . . . is so great that, within a year, half the population has left the neighborhood and has been replaced" (Eyre, 1979, p. 96). Many who came to the city to escape the supervision of overbearing parents or grandparents retained their rural ways and beliefs, which made them easy victims for *samfi* men. Others returned to small towns or rural homes because of increased food prices. As one young girl with two babies remarked, it was impossible to remain in Kingston after the price of a water coconut reached 12 cents. Any increase in the price of condensed milk (a staple in the island) usually makes headlines in the *Daily Gleaner*.

A sense of transience is reinforced by the need to send young, often unintended, and sometimes unwanted, children back to be reared by rural relatives, and by the frequency with which men find it necessary to leave the city and their mates as work becomes available in the countryside. Among the factors pulling able-bodied men back to rural areas are the bauxite mining and processing operations. This pattern of internal movement often permits private concerns to be masked by the public announcement that it is necessary to leave the city in order to work.

The Boundaries

Kingston Parish is enclosed by the rough horseshoe shape of St. Andrew Parish. Together they form most of the Kingston Metro-

politan Area, the KMA. In the highlands north of the city forming
its main arc, St. Andrew is separated from Portland to the east
and St. Mary to the west by the Grand Ridge of the Blue Mountains. From these airy heights, with their tiny hamlets and home-
steads half hidden from winding, gravel roads by banana fronds
and poinsettia, St. Andrew descends in a few miles from a rural
to an urban setting. Its border with Kingston Parish divides the
KMA into northern and southern halves. Below this point it descends south toward the harbor. The western segment of lower
St. Andrew and Kingston contains residential communities occupied by the new middle class, characteristically punctuated by
pockets of shanties and squatters. The eastern segment, in the
hills, includes Gordon Town and Irish Town, with socioeconomically mixed populations near the University of the West Indies.
These areas appeal to many of Kingston's small but active community of artists, writers, and academicians. Here they live near
long-established families who can depend on each other for personal support in times of stress and who represent to their poorer
neighbors sources of employment, gifts upon the birth of children
or holidays, and influence with authorities when necessary.

On a high ridge immediately overlooking the center city is the
neighborhood of Beverly Hills with the opulent homes and swimming pools of the business rich.

The far western prong of the St. Andrew horseshoe descends
from Spanish Town along the Salt River and is crossed by the
broad, potholed asphalt Marcus Garvey Drive near the Esso re-
finery at the edge of the harbor. Hunt's Bay is visible across the
smoldering dump along the causeway from Garvey Drive to Port
Henderson. In the early 1970s Independence City, a new development at the Port Henderson end of the causeway, was occupied,
and the lights from its rows of boxlike houses, sunbaked and arid
during the day, glimmer across the dark harbor at night. Before
the development the area was known as a hiding place for petty
criminals. It is still the site of small beach restaurants where city
dwellers go on weekends to eat "fry fish," "curry goat," and
"bammy," a dense, unleavened, unsalted bread made from
cassava.

The eastern prong of the St. Andrew horseshoe descends sharply southward to the coast where it extends approximately 11 miles southeast to the border of St. Thomas at the hamlet of Bull Bay.

Below central St. Andrew and between its descending prongs, central Kingston Parish contains most of the old town and many of the older, slowly deteriorating, lower-class neighborhoods closer to the harbor. It also includes the major squares, markets, government buildings, and the newer harborside developments.

Kingston as a Place

The foreign observer and educated Jamaican know Kingston as the chief manufacturing site and the political, economic, and financial seat of the nation, the largest English-speaking city in the Caribbean, with the seventh largest harbor in the world. Kingston's population more than doubled between 1943 and 1970, mainly from internal migration. It has grown, however, without the industrialization characterizing most large migratory terminals in the developing world. Kingston has a persistent fragmented rural character that reminds the migrants of home. In the harbor freighters ride at anchor; across the water from the Palisadoes peninsula which protects the harbor from the open sea one can see the hotels and business buildings of New Kingston, halfway up the slope of the Liguana Plain toward the Mona Hills. The great grey piles of a new mall, built to stimulate overseas trade and bring more tourism to the capital, rise by the water's edge. But the metropolitan area retains many aspects of a dusty, amorphous, vastly overgrown country town. Goats run freely on busy streets, with a wary eye for automobiles and buses. They feed on garbage piled near morning markets or left uncollected by doorsteps. In old, rundown areas they may be joined by chickens or hogs. In the quiet, well-to-do residential neighborhoods up the hill toward Mona, driveways are protected by cattle guards as cows of landless owners graze the grass strips along the street and nibble at plants protruding from walled gardens. Unoccupied territories in residential and industrial areas are vulnerable to squatters, and colonies sometimes appear almost overnight. The squatters often keep pigs, easier to handle and raise than cattle. Because they have no land and do not produce enough waste of their own to feed them, these people arise early in the morning and drive their animals through the colorful gardens of more affluent householders. Battles against roving animals are constant, and many householders post "Bad Dog" signs to ward off the animals' masters.

This is only one aspect of the tension between socioeconomic classes that pervades the city. Lack of meaningful work engenders hopelessness and massive frustration in young men; the noise and crowding of their living quarters contribute to the popularity of rum shops, betting shops, street corners, and back yards as places to congregate, drink, and play dominoes. Sometimes the young men fight with fists, chairs, clubs, bottles, and ratchet knives; getting "wired up" is easy if someone says something "personal" in a situation in which "you feel like you mus' take it out on someone." Guns, too, are used and when the police come they "never hesitate, mon, to use their weapons." The oldest and most influential newspaper, the *Daily Gleaner*, and the tabloid *Star* are filled daily with accounts of muggings, assaults, and housebreakings. Every issue of the *Gleaner* contains stories of attack and death by knife, machete, or gun at the hands of individuals or groups, often for trivial robberies or no discernible reason. Nowhere in the metropolitan area do the middle and upper classes feel safe from some type of attack by the lower, "criminal" class. Heavy grillwork encases the patios and windows of their homes; Kingston's population of large dogs, kept mainly because of the fear of burglary and assault, produces a nightly background of barks and howls audible in the otherwise quiet hills above the central city. In 1974 so many upper-class and political figures were shot that the government established a gun court with indefinite sentences for illegal possession of arms. This enclosure of barbed wire and watch towers remains, a new landmark for Kingstonians.

Some migrants from the country remain in the transitional slums; others eventually move to more stable high- or medium-density neighborhoods or to peripheral shantytowns. Kingston's built-up areas include approximately 40 square miles traversed by tightly packed buses, private cars, taxis, "robots" (local varieties of private jitney), motorcycles, donkey carts, bicycles, and people on foot. The localities whose names end in *Town*, such as Denham Town or Trenchtown, are often lower-class areas with inadequate municipal services. The word *Pen*, an old English term, originally designated a small village grouped around a cattle pen. When Prime Minister Hugh Shearer introduced the first electric generator to the village of Hunt's Pen in December 1971, he humorously remarked, "Now that Hunt's Pen has electricity you'll be sending a deputation asking me to change the name to Hunt's Town". (In the same speech he is also reported to have predicted that with the advent of electricity the village birthrate would decline.) Many Kingston streets, especially in the downtown area, are called lanes—Rum Lane, Love Lane, Honeysuckle Lane, Bread Lane, Chapel Lane, Widow's Lane—the old term for an unpaved alley between rows of mean houses, with a disparaging connotation. One resident magistrate in Kingston betrayed his assumptions about petty criminals when he asked the man in the dock before him what lane he lived in.

The original business district has lost its function as the center of town except for the poorer people. Accessibility is also reduced by traffic congestion. The rapid proliferation of shopping plazas in more recently developed residential areas "uptown," toward the hills, has led to further abandonment of the downtown area by middle-class Kingstonians, especially at night. Thus, the old town center, inadequately lit and increasingly far from home, tends to be left to its lower-class and transitional inhabitants. Increasing crime and violence have contributed to this desertion. Middle-class Kingstonians go there reluctantly, even for the popular pantomime performances at the Ward Theatre; and if they do visit this theatre, they make sure to pay some local entrepreneur 50 cents for "minding" their car during the performance to be sure of finding it intact afterward.

Nevertheless, patients from these poor sections displayed a sense of home and physical belonging in the sureness and confidence with which they guided me through the labyrinthine pathways to their shanties or between deteriorating buildings and across poorly defined yards. They greeted others with increasing frequency as we approached the core of the home area. A young-ster leaning against a corrugated tin fence testing the blade of a ratchet knife or machete with his thumb would be noted and passed in quick silence. They also registered unfamiliar faces: "Me not know him. Wonder who he looking for?"

Residential Patterns

The most commonly referred to social dividing points in Kings-ton are Cross Roads and Half Way Tree, close to each other in lower St. Andrew and linked by the Half Way Tree Road. Origi-nally a market where traffic centered around the weekly influx of higglers (independent country vendors) and their customers, Cross Roads is roughly halfway between the upper border of Kingston Parish (marked by the racetrack) and the New Kingston development. Spectacular growth has occurred there since 1960 and retail volume along Half Way Tree Road north on Cross Roads is estimated to exceed that of the downtown area. Choked with people, cars, handcart men, buses, and fumes, the section of Half Way Tree around and above Cross Roads has few foreign visitors except those securely encased in their automobiles en route down to the government buildings and harbor or up to New Kingston and the residential areas in the hills.

Also common are references to living "above" or "below" the Clock, a clocktower built at the junction of Hope and Constant Spring roads during the celebration of Queen Victoria's Jubilee, when many similar ones were installed at village crossroads throughout the island. "Above the Clock" lies most of New Kings-ton, the site of the golf club, embassies, the residences of the prime minister and governor-general amid extensive gardens, and glossy hotels occupied by visiting businessmen and tourists on one- or two-day conducted excursions. Their bars, restau-rants, and swimming pools serve as informal clubs for the local and moderately well-to-do middle class. New Kingston is also a place of banks, duty-free shops, and restaurants built to take advantage of what was hoped to become a greatly expanded stream of commercial visitors and tourists. This is the area in which upwardly mobile and urbanized low-class Kingstonians, touts and *samfi* men living by their wits, attempt contact with foreign visitors, offering themselves as drivers, guides, prostitutes, or purveyors of rare goods including ganja, or selling jewelry, clothing, or food on streetcorners. Here, too, are the old upperclass residential area of Vale Royal and newer middle-class condominiums and townhouses. But even here, just off the main streets, the visitor may unexpectedly encounter a cow or goat. Nowhere are residential sections homogeneous: even "above" the Clock and Cross Roads there are large pockets of shanties and semiurbanized squatters' homes extending along the gullies, open sewers, and drains.

"Below" the Clock the neighborhoods become increasingly, though not uniformly, ill-kempt. Neat homes of civil servants and clerks, a developing lower-middle class, are found on some streets, but behind stucco walls deceptively bright with scarlet poinsettia and lavender bougainvillea, streets running parallel to Half Way Tree often conceal dusty yards with multifamily dwellings, indicated by fractional street numbers and clusters of mailboxes at the gate. Goats nudge uncollected garbage, and although occasional cars park along streets without sidewalks, the traffic is mainly pedestrian.

Farther down toward the harbor are Trench Town and Tivoli Gardens, the former "dungle" (a local perversion of *jungle*) where people combed the garbage dumps for food, now rebuilt with modern flats and small parks. The subcommunities here are regularly described by the sober, employed, lower-middle class as the homes of "bad men," "men with guns," and "gangs" of criminals. Townspeople living elsewhere perceive them as jealously guarded territories, strongholds to which the government is reluctant to send inspectors for normal municipal surveys and services. In recent years this has also become true for some of the shantytowns near Kingston; knowledgeable Family Planning Clinic personnel stated with conviction that any stranger, Jamaican or otherwise, will be met with hostility in these neighborhoods, which contain many unemployed persons and "Rastas."

The Rastafarians, especially the most visibly striking "locks-men," are often viewed with suspicion and fear because of their unkempt hair and beards, their dissociation from the conventional capitalist world of Jamaica, and their use of ganja.

Many of the old middle-class residential areas below the Clock have become homes for the working class or unemployed. In 1968 these neighborhoods accounted for 42.5 percent of a representative Kingston population (Norton, 1974, 1978). Several estimates suggest that this area, including the slum of West Kingston, now contains at least half the KMA population. Those areas adjacent to high-density slums, in a constant process of invasion by lower-income people, show signs of deterioration with neglected grounds, multiple-family occupancy, pit toilets, and nonresidential use, including tailor shops, rum shops, barbers, automobile repair yards, and small industries. Temporary structures often house additional people or provide cooking space. In the more affluent areas, small apartments or cottages constructed for rental often occupy the grounds of original dwellings. Some buildings retaining signs of Victorian elegance have become tenements, with their grounds converted into yards. In the older sections with buildings mainly constructed prior to 1942, rum shops, eating places, and food shops are commonly grouped in small clusters of corner stores that form the foci of neighborhoods. Many are marginal operations dealing in very small quantities, giving credit to customers, and frequently changing hands. Here, too, are small, shabby hotels, including some used for sexual intercourse with prostitutes and pickups, and commercial lodging houses. This transitional zone contains rows of slum tenements that provide the first housing for incoming rural migrants. Here, it is popularly said, 'Two hundred people move each night." In one neighborhood, Jonestown (Gentles, 1968), 80 percent of the householders were born outside the metropolitan area and 31 percent had moved five or more times, usually within the area.

In these dwellings crowding is a common feature. The 1973 sample survey of central Kingston revealed an average density of 3.6 persons per room, with 77 percent of householders being tenants, 14 percent squatters, and only 9 percent owner-occupiers

(Norton, 1978). Especially notable is the pressure for sleeping space: a tiny room is commonly filled by two double beds side by side, with no room for additional furniture. Some tiny houses may contain a mixture of wood, formica, and plastic furniture, and often a transistor radio or television set. The places for cooking, laundering, excreting, and socializing are in the yard (shared with members of other families) or under corrugated tin, cardboard, canvas, or scrapwood lean-tos against the main structure.

The housing context in which our respondents, informants, and their neighbors lived is suggested by the 1970 census data: in central Kingston only 14 percent of all dwellings had water piped into the building and in 66,000 households an outside pipe was shared with others; toilet facilities were shared with other family groups in 80 percent of all Kingston households; and 43 percent of all dwellings in Kingston and St. Andrew consisted of only one room (Eyre, 1979).

Shantytowns

Shantytowns housed 22.8 percent of Norton's representative housing survey of the KMA in 1968 (1974). Few of these dwellings have piped water; when they do it is usually by illegal connection to a main. In many cases a single standpipe open for only a few hours daily serves several hundred people. There are no street lights, drainage, or garbage collection. The open sewers, increasing the likelihood of disease, are vulnerable to floods and hurricanes. The majority of toilets are pits. The location of just under 50 percent of the island's "rent-free dwellings" in the KMA suggests that many are built by squatters on land so far unclaimed or ignored by government or private owners (1970 Census, Bulletin 2, 1973).

Shantytown dwellers are a fertile population. In the largest shantytown of Montego Bay the average number of children under age four per 100 women aged 15 to 44 was 72, compared with 53 per 100 in the rest of the city (Eyre, 1976). This may be related to the more balanced sex ratio (113 to 120 females per 100 males) in the shantytowns than in the urban area as a whole, where (although females constitute only 51 percent of the census

population) there are some census tracts with more than 150 females for every 100 males. The St. James Family Planning Association, part of JFPA, operates a free clinic in Montego Bay,
where almost one-fifth of the women from two studied shantytowns were registered in 1970, but despite intensified contraception campaigns there was little increase in participation between
then and 1974.

In the KMA heavy concentrations of shantytowns are found to
the west along Spanish Town Road, parallel to the harbor; to the
east on the edges of the metropolitan area, as in Long Mountain
and the Wareika Hills, known as refuges for petty criminals, Rastafarians, and ganja dealers; and, as previously noted, in occupied pockets of land, along gullies, and near river beds throughout the area.

The Clinic Populations and Their Neighborhoods

East Street, site of the major Jamaica Family Planning Association clinic, is a mixed residential and business neighborhood in
the heart of the old city, Kingston Parish, located far below Cross
Roads. Many of the clients, especially men, come because it is
convenient to their place of work. Men and women also attend
this clinic at a distance from their homes because it offers a degree of anonymity; several women said that it was less crowded
than the Victoria Jubilee Hospital and that they preferred it because it was "not a hospital."

Female clients were registered according to home address.
Approximately two-thirds came from the old high-density, transitional neighborhoods, mainly the more stable, long-settled areas
that altogether account for approximately 60 percent of the KMA
population. The rest were fairly evenly distributed among new
high-density, medium-density, and low-density areas. None lived
in an identifiable shantytown. Most were of non-Kingston origin
(50 percent rural and 26 percent from small towns) and only a
few of these had been reared in the city.

The Manley Clinic, where the noncontraceptive users were
interviewed, is located on Grant's Pen Road in a semirural slum

below the Barbican business area and somewhat above Cross Roads and the Clock. This is a lower-class neighborhood of long-settled St. Andrew with mixed residential and small business pockets, shantytown clumps in the vicinity, and some nearby high-density housing. The residences of its patients were scattered between old low-density and new high- and medium-density areas. Some lived in nearby shantytowns. Others came up from the transitional and other high-density areas of Kingston Parish.

Table 1 shows a comparison of the housing conditions of the respondents with the conditions of the KMA as a whole. The combined JFPA and Manley client-patient resembled the mean Kings-

Table 1. Housing characteristics of respondents in 1974 and of KMA population in 1970,[a] in percentages.

Housing characteristics	150 women[b]	283 men[c]	KMA dwellings
Type			
Single room or tenement	57.3	30.0	44.0
Detached house or conventional apartment	42.7	70.0	—[d]
Utilities			
Inside electricity	78.7	97.9	—[e]
Inside piped water	46.0[f]	81.3	43.0
Inside toilet	44.7	81.6	—[g]

a. KMA data compiled from *Jamaica population census, 1970*, Bulletin 2 (Kingston: Jamaica Department of Statistics, 1973).

b. Of 100 JFPA clients and 50 nonclients, no women lived alone. No residential mobility data were obtained.

c. All the men were JFPA clients. Of these, 9.2 percent lived alone; 39.1 percent had changed residence 4-8 times and 33.7 percent 1-3 times since arriving in Kingston; 91.5 percent had not moved in the year preceding the interview.

d. Census data are not applicable because they include one-room houses and apartments.

e. Not recorded in census.

f. Only 23.3 percent of Manley Clinic contraceptive never-users had piped water.

g. This figure, though not recorded in the census, is limited by the availability of piped water and must therefore be less than 43 percent. Water closets (in contrast with pits), including shared ones in the yard, were recorded for 82 percent of the dwellings.

tonian in terms of amenities (represented by inside piped water) but had less living space, due mainly to the prevalence of one-room dwellings among the 77 percent of Manley Clinic never-users of rural origin. No woman or her mate from either population owned the dwelling; none of the women and only 12 of their mates (8 percent) owned land "in the country."

In most cases, for the more than half of urban households without interior plumbing, a standpipe in the yard, generally used by several families, provided water. Most of the rest depended on a standpipe at a public place such as a streetcorner. The incongruities between the failure to supply half the population with adequate plumbing and easily available water for drinking and washing, the lack of privacy, and the expectation that people living in such surroundings would effectively use sophisticated contraceptive technology were acknowledged by only a few family planning administrators and personnel with whom I talked. These features, along with lack of privacy in the clinics and insufficient counseling services, are part of the institutional context in which individual use or nonuse of contraceptive methods must be understood.

5 Women without Power: The Social and Economic Context of Sex and Reproduction

Woman a ebby load, woman a ebby load
Woman a ebby load, when Satiday mawning come

When de money no 'nough, when de money no 'nough
When de money no 'nough, dem call yu john crow man

But when de money 'nough, when de money 'nough
When de money 'nough, dem call yu sweety pie

Why woman grumble so, wan' more money
Why woman grumble so, wan' more money

Dem get it dem grumble, wan' more money
Dem no get it dem grumble, wan' more money
Mek promise dem grumble, wan' more money

> *Recorded in rural Jamaica and reproduced*
> *with the permission of Olive Lewin*

In Jamaica . . . we are today reaping the results, in crime, unemployment and illiteracy, of over-breeding in the past . . . It is not just a matter of food. It is also a matter of the quality of life.

> *Thomas Wright, in the* Daily Gleaner
> *Kingston, 22 March 1975*

It was hard with my mother having all of us. Especially to find meat and clothes.

> *A woman at the East Street clinic*

Statistical data on reproductively active Jamaicans and those who are less so suggest that certain aspects of sexual-reproductive activity are associated with particular socioeconomic and demographic factors. It does not, however, follow that any of these factors are necessary, unique, or sufficient causes or reasons for the behaviors in question. Nor are the percentages of variance that can be attributed to one or another factor valid for an understanding of the whole person whose behavior is being examined. With these reservations the following pages present the significance of several such factors for sexual-reproductive behavior, including attempts to manage one's own fertility. In particular, education, traditional beliefs, and urban birth, even within this predominantly working-class group, are associated with resistance or conformity to the pronatal pressures within the society. These characteristics, presented in terms both of the sample population size and of correlations with aspects of sexual-reproductive behavior, are relevant for the island as a whole to the degree that the respondents' socioeconomic status and demographic characteristics can be systematically related to those of Jamaicans in general.

Socioeconomic and Sexual Powerlessness

It is easy for a middle-class North American, confronted with a Brazilian *favelada* or a Jamaican pregnant without financial support, to conclude that she does not plan for the future; a psychologist might remark that she is not "future oriented" or does not value independence, personal autonomy, or upward mobility. Our Jamaican respondents were in fact intensely sensitive to what they and their children might achieve and to what their lives would be like in their old age. But for those who must constantly cope with an overwhelming present, the boundary between what is personal and what is economic often remains undefined. Survival on the continuing edge of disaster demands attention to concrete immediacies. Lack of resources, opportunity, and knowledge, a sense of frustrated aspirations, and a frequent sense of being discriminated against weigh heavily in their awareness. Their distrust of presumably helping authority has become chronic. In the 1960s most men felt themselves unfairly treated by bosses and 84 percent preferred a different kind of work (Netherlands, 1968). In the 1970s most of our female respondents said of their employers, "Them not treat me right." Under these circumstances lack of energy and resources to delay present gratification for future gain is complicated by doubt that those "on top" will let them change their lives. The anger of the poorest people tends to be submerged in apathy. It is expressed for them by those who are talented and have made it upward, especially in the music called *reggae*. Reggae in Jamaica is often the vehicle for social protest. Recent songs of Marcia Griffith and Bob Marley, for example, speak of survival, and of the anger of the oppressed people toward the few "on top" who control them.

The authority that urges birth control may be similarly suspect even when economically marginal people understand and mourn their inability to care adequately for their children. It is, after all, "the control" that they perceive as pressed upon them. Ambivalence seems heightened by family planning advertising that emphasizes the importance of being able to support the children one brings into the world. The implication is clear: people with enough money can have the children they want; it is only the poor who must be "controlled."

Moreover, the contraceptive message is based on a middle-class family image derived from the white, British-European culture, from industrial societies with low infant mortality in which children are not potential sources of social and economic support and in which a small family means more money for consumer goods. Jamaica's infant mortality rate in 1970, at 33 per 1,000 for females and 37 for males, was approximately three times that of European and North American levels; limited available data suggest that it did not change significantly in the ensuing ten years. This message advises the use of technical, scientific methods to influence a natural function highly valued by traditional peoples. As such, it is directed to a group still unprepared to receive it: the least educated, underemployed majority, sympathetic to non-technical healing systems. In terms of values and attitudes these people are part of a rural traditional society maintaining coexistence with one that is urban and modern. Old traditions, expressed in the attitudes and behavior of country folk, coexist with the technical, future-directed outlook orienting the educated, economically dominant, though numerically small elite. This situation exists in many former plantation societies, but the government family planning campaign in Jamaica emphasizes the incongruity between traditional and modern in a particular way that is also potentially coercive. On one hand, men and women and their children have the right to information and services essential to reproductive self-determination. On the other, the very force and ubiquitousness of the contraceptive message seems at times to militate against its reflective use by individuals and couples.

The anger that might arise in this situation does not surface in interviews with a physician. Perhaps the women are not themselves conscious of any anger. Trapped in a system that does not allow them the resources to care for the children they want, they must apply to the same system for devices that interfere with their natural fertility. Their ambivalence is suggested by the vagueness of their answers to questions about why they have not previously taken advantage of the widely advertised and nearby contraceptive services. Ambivalence also seems reflected in the frequency with which contraceptive use, once started, is abandoned.

When, early in my stay on the island, I saw the frustration of Jamaican colleagues pursuing clear answers to what appeared to be clear questions, I felt that they lacked interviewing skills. Later I found myself confronted with the same vagueness, however masked in apparent compliance. One oppressive morning when the small office fan hardly evaporated the film of sweat on my face, I began to experience an impatience bordering on anger. The young woman sitting in the room with me in the East Street clinic seemed amiable and cooperative, but I felt I was being deliberately frustrated. Once I was aware of the feeling, it was replaced by a sense of the two of us as components of a single process; my incipient anger might be the conscious reflection of something present in her but outside her awareness. Then I remembered an expression I had already heard several times— "the pressure," a constant tension from which there is no escape.

At that moment I was feeling the same pressure. I decided to ask the woman about it.

I said, "Sometimes the pressure gets pretty heavy, doesn't it?" She seemed startled. Her friendly smile disappeared, but only for seconds. She replied, "They say better soon come, pressure drop, but hard to know." Still the interview really was not turned around. She could not get beyond an "I don't know" as a reason for not having come to the clinic before having, at age 23, three children by two men neither of whom was contributing to her support. But as she talked of her sense of personal isolation in Kingston her anger and disappointment at the second man, who had promised "to care me and my child," and the difficulties of survival in the city, her "I don't know" emerged as an expression of paralysis. Beaten down by "the pressure," she might think a solution existed in "having a baby for" a man who could "care" her. If he failed to do so, having babies might be a way of constructing her own group for herself. But without money this process would be self-defeating; she would have to give away the babies she produced to be reared by others. Family planning was a source of hope, but "the control" was foreign and possibly dangerous. For her, I thought, it might represent less a move toward personal autonomy than submitting to the system and precluding her natural way of affirming herself. For this woman without education or a personal support system, already responsible for three new lives that she had conceived, it would have been stranger, more unexpected, to have come up with a rational reason for delaying contraceptive use than to have said simply and authentically that she did not know the reason.

"The pressure" has also been incorporated into reggae. F. Hibbert's song "Pressure Drop" states "Pressure gonna drop on you . . . When it drops oh you gotta feel it/Know that you were doin' wrong." "The pressure" includes not only economic oppression from above but also victimization by other poor people as the threat of theft and assault becomes part of the slumdweller's ordinary experience. It is also associated with sex and reproduction. The feeling of helplessness is expressed with particular emphasis by women with young children whose care limits their mobility and employment opportunities. They cannot count on their conjugal partners' consistent support even on Saturday morning, the time to market for food for the coming week. Many suspect their men of parasitic tendencies and go to some lengths to hide whatever earnings they do have: "Them not want to work . . . just jig and jig . . . and then them want you to feed them." There is little sharing of information about money. Instead, an attitude of cautious, protective wariness prevails. As one woman said of her current partner, "Sometimes him bad and keep it all to himself." Many note that their men want to keep them pregnant so as to prevent their going with others but are unwilling to support them. They feel that this is unfair. As one said, "If him want to keep me for himself, him just need care me. But him wants his money so can have others too."

The tendency to view sexual partners as part of an essentially exploitative socioeconomic system is not confined to women of the lowest socioeconomic status. One young secretary in a hotel with many foreign guests spoke bitterly of her boy friend, one of its junior managers: "He gets angry if a customer wants to take me out just because he wants to be sure he can do it with me any time he feels like it. If I don't feel like it, he gets mad and goes off to see his girl friend up on Stony Hill." The bargaining aspects of sex are acknowledged even by the middle class. As an educated Jamaican woman, divorced and alone for several years, told me one evening, "I've had my children and I don't need men any more. If a man wants to sleep with me he will have to buy me a house in the hills!"

The Vulnerability of Children and Mothers

Without other opportunities for self-expression or ego extension and with few social or economic resources, men and women try to achieve them through parenthood and having children. But pleasure in parenthood is diminished by awareness that the long-range promise of a child's companionship in old age is uncertain. More important is the brutal impact of poverty, which denies parents and children the most primitive capacity for environmental control. Awareness of vulnerability to external forces as a result of inadequate food and shelter is intensified by awareness of lack of knowledge—as one woman said, about "how things run."

The realities of lower-class Jamaican children and their parents are clear in the government's own statements about nutrition, housing, schooling, and employment. "For children under three years of age there is a serious deficiency in protein intake . . . Malnutrition and gastroenteritis combined are the most common causes of death in this age group . . . 85 percent of children up to six years of age receive less than the minimum desirable requirement of calories" (CPU, 1970-1975, Part III, Section C, p. 6).

In the central slums of Kingston 200 to 400 people per acre occupy private dwellings intermingled with industrial and commercial buildings. As surrounding development land is sold, low-income families become progressively more cramped and the "core slum" spreads by the "breaking down of the edges of adjoining areas into twilight slums" incorporating older residential suburbs (CPU, 1970-1975, Part III, Section D5, p. 4).

Jamaican educators have attributed the country's problems in social development in part to its lack of an effective system of public education (Figueroa, 1971). Inability to read and write, estimated by various sources at up to 50 percent of the adult population, was of sufficient public concern in 1974 to warrant a literacy campaign. Official reports state that existing schools and teachers are inadequate to the task: "The quality of education received by the pupils is seriously deficient" (Ministry of Education, 1973, p. 14). In the primary schools "the system is critically handicapped by irregularity of attendance, gross overcrowding, vestigial equipment and instructional materials and inadequate numbers of teachers, trained and untrained. Conditions are so primitive that the mind boggles at the thought of the conditions under which teachers must teach and children learn" (p. 14). Three-fourths of the respondents had not gone beyond primary school, a proportion comparable with that of other women in the Kingston-St. Andrew area (table 2). These tend to be the younger

Table 2. Educational level of Jamaicans, in percentages.[a]

Educational level	General population male and female, 14 years and over (N = 1,009,690)[b]	Labor force male and female, 14 years and over (N = 577,039)[c]	Kingston-St. Andrew females 7 years and over (N = 216,505)[d]	Study population Kingston-St. Andrew females 16 years and over (N = 150)
No schooling	3.9	3.3	—	1.3
Incomplete primary	34.1	8.6	—	12.0
Complete primary[e]	52.7	71.5	—	62.7
Some or complete primary	86.8	80.1	77.0	74.7
Some or complete secondary	7.7	11.0	19.8	18.0
Technical/commercial	0.8	4.0	2.0	5.3
Some or complete university	0.5	1.0	1.2	0.7
Beyond primary	9.0	16.0	23.0	24.0

a. All but the fourth column are computed from *Jamaica population census, 1970*, Bulletin 3 (Kingston: Jamaica Department of Statistics, 1974). Census data exclude 56,489 persons residing in institutions or with incomplete data.

b. Only 9.3 percent of the population aged 14 and above are still in school.

c. Excludes 9,406 people with incomplete data.

d. Includes all still attending primary school and above. Excludes 20,980 in nursery/infant schools, 38,524 with no years of education, and 1,489 with incomplete data. Assumed to include mainly those aged 7 and above, both attending and finished with school. Those listed as having no education are assumed to be mainly below age 7, but 1-2 percent, in keeping with other data, may be aged 14 or older, which would reduce the educated percentage.

e. Primary schooling in the census data referred to only 5 years.

women, and age is negatively correlated with educational achievement (gamma −.43). Approximately 13 percent had a fourth-grade education or less, and more than one-fifth could no more than read or write their name and make change.

Secondary high schools have admitted only about 8 percent of the appropriate age group: "The school system is dominated by a series of examinations which are . . . notable for their failure rate, limit the curriculum . . . and engender boredom and dislike of learning, particularly in the secondary schools" (p. 5).

Being without work means not only economic deprivation but also lack of an important source of self-esteem that leads eventually to passivity and apathy. Official estimates of unemployment in 1972 (National Planning Agency) averaged 22.8 percent. Unofficial estimates in 1975 ranged from one-fourth to one-third of the labor force, with the figure for less than full-time employment as much as 50 percent or higher. Even this may be low, depending on how many people are regarded as part of the labor force. Young men tend to be less fully employed than their elders. Women are even more irregularly employed, but more often have jobs as, with increasing age, they are relieved from childbearing and child care. In the Kingston Metropolitan Area 73.5 percent of females, approximately the same number as the 74.5 percent of males past age 14, were employed either part- or full-time during the study period (Department of Statistics, Bulletin 5, 1974). A review of national labor data showed the main categories of "skilled" employment available to women to be weaving straw and making dresses (Francis, 1973). The main sources of employment were domestic. Of the 150 female respondents two-thirds (table 3), reflecting the demands of child care that keep them at home, were employed at least part-time. Of these the largest number, 41, were unskilled manual workers including domestics, who along with another 23 factory workers (including many cigar makers) and drivers (classed as skilled) made up almost two-thirds of the employed group. They reported 94.6 percent of their mates as employed full- or part-time. This figure, higher than those of the census, probably reflects the male partner's somewhat greater age as well as the women's lack of detailed knowl-

Table 3. Employment and occupation of 150 Jamaican women and their mates, in percentages.

Employment status	Women	Mates
Employed at least part-time[a]	66.3 (73.5)[b]	94.6 (74.5)[b]
Manual, unskilled[c]	27.3	16.0
Manual, skilled[d]	15.3	46.7
Nonmanual[e]	24.0	32.0
Never employed	23.3	00.0

a. Includes some also housewives and students.

b. According to *Jamaica population census, 1970,* Bulletin 5 (Kingston, Department of Statistics, 1974), for the week preceding census day the total labor force for Jamaica was 378,288 males and 188,157 females, with 81.6 and 75.9 percent, respectively, employed, part-time or full-time. For the combined Kingston-St. Andrew area the figures were 109,446 males and 81,820 females, with 74.5 and 73.5 percent, respectively, employed part-time or full-time. Employment figures were calculated from numbers "not applicable" or "classified." The data do not permit calculation of skilled and unskilled manual or nonmanual categories.

c. Includes domestics, custodial workers, and higglers.

d. Includes factory operatives, fishermen, carpenters, and drivers.

e. Includes clerical, skilled white-collar, and minor executive roles.

edge of the actual economic status of their visiting partners. Approximately two-thirds of the male partners of these women appeared to be manual, mainly unskilled, workers.

It is evident that this is a society with few viable economic roles for either men or women, and probable that in such a context child producing and rearing offer significant possibilities for status and self-affirmation, especially to women. One study of "higglering" (taking country produce to sell in city markets) suggests that female work roles have lower status and rewards, even when they are as economically productive as those of men or more so (Durant-Gonzales, 1976). A 1973 sample survey of central Kingston found that approximately half the average household incomes came from absent fathers for the support of their children (Norton, 1978). In such mother-headed households, which constitute a large proportion of those in the metropolitan area, women are captive to the needs of their children, angrily dependent upon and often contemptuous of the frequent capriciousness of men "for whom" they "had the babies" in helping support them. They perceive Jamaican men simultaneously as weaklings and as oppressors who undeservedly occupy more advantaged positions (see chapter 8).

The Female Respondents

Selection by Pregnancy and Contraceptive Status

The 50 JFPA clients called "early users" (those with zero to two pregnancies) include 15 who were never pregnant. Three of these were first-time attendees. One was a 16-year-old who, after regular intercourse for three months with one partner, decided she was "not ready to have a baby." Her partner had made the decision for her to use a technical method rather than for him to use a condom. One was an 18-year-old who had not yet had intercourse and wanted to be protected before she did. The partner with whom she planned to have sexual relations felt negative about her decision. The third woman was a 28-year-old, celibate for a long period because of her beliefs as a Jehovah's Witness. She had had approximately nine months of regular intercourse before stopping, and came now for contraceptive services prior to marriage. The decision was hers, but her fiancé agreed.

The other 12 never-pregnant clients had also engaged in intercourse, but hoped, they said, to delay their first pregnancy. The partner of one 19-year-old with 24 months of regular intercourse had used withdrawal (coitus interruptus) for nine months before asking her to come to JFPA. One 23-year-old with 30 months of regular intercourse with two partners had used a variety of technical methods before coming to the clinic. Of all the others who had had intercourse before coming to JFPA, a 25-year-old had had intercourse for the longest period, 46 months. It seems likely that many of these women had avoided pregnancy less because of contraception than because of fertility impaired by disease or other factors. Also, their decision to begin contraception even though they had not conceived seemed to reflect less need to affirm their status and self-esteem through child production. This factor was congruent with their relatively advantaged status.

Their mean age at the time of interview was 20, compared with a mean age of 26 for those having been pregnant at least once. Almost three times as many (48 versus 16 percent) had been born in Kingston, and twice as many (59 versus 27 percent) had gone beyond sixth grade. Another indication of more socioeconomically privileged backgrounds was the fact that more (65 versus 44 percent) lived in homes with piped water. All aspired to upward mobility and most were already engaged in nonmanual work. Whether the aspirations antedated initial intercourse or whether they developed because the women were able to continue in school is uncertain. It is possible that freedom from pregnancy and child care (which so often burdened their peers) permitted them greater self-determination and ambition.

Of 22 sexually active and not contracepting Manley Clinic patients with zero to two pregnancies, two, aged 17 and 21, had never been pregnant despite eight months of regular intercourse. Together these two groups contained 72 women, almost half (48 percent) of the total respondents, with a relatively limited experience of the reproductive consequences of intercourse.

The other 52 percent of the 150 respondents included 50 JFPA "late users," with three to ten pregnancies at the time of the research interview, and 28 Manley Clinic nonusers with the same number of pregnancies. Approximately half of these 78 women had been pregnant five or more times. Twenty of the 50 Manley Clinic nonusers had terminated earlier brief periods of contraception in order to conceive or, having conceived despite contraception, had not resumed it. Thus, these were women with significantly more experience of the reproductive consequences of intercourse.

Only 6 percent of the entire group of 133 women ever pregnant had used contraception prior to their first pregnancy, 16.6 percent prior to their second pregnancy. Furthermore, the idea of being a contraceptive "user" is misleading in its implication of consistency. For most respondents, use of contraceptives had been haphazard; only 56 of the 130 who had ever used a method said they had started and stopped use in accordance with conscious intentions. Of the 85 current users with children, 35 said they hoped to space future births and the remaining 50 said they wanted no more children. Only 28 of the 85, however, had ever used a method for as long as four months. It is not surprising, then, that having zero to two in contrast to three to ten pregnancies is significantly correlated with age (gamma .76, table 4). It reflects for the first group fewer years of sexual exposure rather than systematic contraceptive use.

This sample suggests the fragile subjective reality of contraceptive use on the island: only 6 percent of the women ever pregnant, regardless of age (gamma .07), had tried to contracept prior to first pregnancy; only one of the women never pregnant had acquired a contraceptive prior to first intercourse. Instead, table 4 indicates an overall positive correlation between age and total number of births (gamma .61), pregnancies (gamma .58), and number of men by whom they have become pregnant (gamma .50). Years of social life after puberty appear for most to mean years of sexual and reproductive life. Fertility is less a function of

Table 4. Gamma correlations of age and indicators of socioeconomic status for 150 Jamaican women.

Indicators	Age	Education	Urban birth	Piped water in home
Age	1.00	−.43	−.27	.08
Education	−.43	1.00	.39	.61
Urban birth	−.27	.39	1.00	.63
Piped water	−.08	.61	.63	1.00
Literacy	−.22	.88	.40	.22
Number of live births	.61	−.50	−.23	−.35
Number of pregnancies	.58	−.47	−.22	−.33
Number of male impregnators	.50	−.55	−.35	−.47
Positive attitude to contraception	.22	.46	.42	.56
Smaller ideal family size	−.18	.36	.09	.13
Discussed contraception with mate	.15	.33	.10	.33
Knowledge of reproductive physiology	.07	.69	.25	.49
Mate's occupational status	−.16	.36	.29	.44
Choice of oral contraceptive	.14	.38	.33	.30
Purposeful contraceptive effort	.04	.60	.47	.57
Contraceptive agreement with partner	−.02	.26	−.04	.42

contraceptive use than of the amount of time available to engage in sexual intercourse.

Age-Related Behaviors and Attitudes and Cultural Change

The 150 women constituted a young population. Their age range was 16 to 47, with 83.4 percent less than 31, 92.1 percent less than 35, and a median of 25.5 years. It is reasonable to assume that their behavior reflects a generational change in the sexual-reproductive culture of the island, whether in connection with the development of public education in general, the dissemination of reproductive knowledge and contraceptive services since 1967-68, continuing migration to other societies—sometimes circular—or worldwide changes in attitudes toward sex and family life. The data, however, do not support this assumption. Rather, they suggest that even for this population oriented to clinics and services, after puberty sexual intercourse and its consequences, pregnancy and childbirth, occur repeatedly and cumulatively. Only one of the 17 never pregnant respondents had attempted to interfere with this sequence by using technical contraceptive methods prior to first intercourse. Only 8 of the 133 ever pregnant women had used such methods prior to first pregnancy, and these were not the youngest. Not until after their third pregnancy did approximately one-fourth begin to try seriously to manage their fertility. On the island as a whole it was estimated that fewer than half of all women between ages 15 and 44 had ever tried a technical method at least once—at any time in their lives (Sinclair, 1974). In 1974, of course, 44-year-old women had had easy access to public clinics only since 1967, when they were 37 years old; family planning services, though, had been available to those who wanted them for years before that time. Furthermore, considering that the median age on the island has remained near 15 for approximately 30 years; that the typical contraceptive seeker has been a woman already burdened with several children; and that birthrates have not changed significantly since the 1960s, it appears doubtful that the highly publicized government program with its greatly increased number of clinics has been a significant factor in delaying first pregnancies or increasing the time between the first and second pregnancies. It is apparent also that those who have sustained a contraceptive effort even for a few months constitute a distinct minority.

Nevertheless, even within this working-class population age is intercorrelated in many ways (table 4) with education, with urban birth, and with more privileged surroundings (indicated by having piped water in the home) and probably higher socioeconomic status. The younger women did not have more adequate dwellings, but all four items are correlated with lower levels of reproductive activity. Moreover, respondents who have never used contraceptives are least likely to have more than a primary education, mates of higher occupational status, and utilities in their homes. The proportion increases from the current nonusers (Manley patients) to current users (JFPA clients).

Given these considerations, the question arises whether cultural change may be reflected more in attitudes and outlook than in actual contraceptive use. The socioeconomic and familial features observed in the 1970s were similar to those reported by investigators in the 1950s. In the 1970s educators still spoke of the "dry years," especially for girls; these were the years between age 14, when those who went to high school (less than one-fourth of the population) had finished, and the time when they could be regarded as sufficiently mature to be employable or to establish households of their own. During these years a major route to self-affirmation as a potential adult and to status in the peer group was through pregnancy.

The younger JFPA clients in particular and the younger women in general, have in fact had more general schooling and more sexual-reproductive education. Younger women are more likely to have obtained sexual-reproductive information from public sources (gamma .43) and to have obtained it earlier from any source (gamma .34). This change does not seem to have penetrated the family, however: younger women have not more significantly received sexual-reproductive information from their mothers. Nor is there a correlation between age and a positive attitude toward contraception, even though a positive attitude would be expected in an early user.

More impressive, however, is the absence of significant correlations between age and a number of fertility-related factors, suggesting that basic cultural change is not reflected in the comparison of younger and older respondents (table 5). Thus, there are no significant differences between younger and older respondents in favoring the traditional role of the grandmother in the family, a belief in the woman's having a foreordained "lot" of children, general knowledge of reproductive physiology, a feeling of primary responsibility to mother and not to mate, favoring a smaller ideal family size, beliefs in bizarre side effects of contraception, more adequate communication with first or coital sexual partners, or memories of verbal rather than physical parental discipline. Some of these indexes are correlated with education rather than with age as such: positive attitudes to contraception, smaller ideal family size, general knowledge of reproductive

Table 5. Gamma correlations of fertility-related factors with age and education for 150 Jamaican women.

Fertility-related factors	Age	Education
Education	−.43	1.00
Earlier sex instruction	−.34	.37
Kingston birth	−.27	.39
Sex information from mother	−.20	.37
Smaller ideal family size	−.18	.36
Positive communication with first coital partner	−.18	.20
Favors traditional grandmother role	.13	−.41
Belief in "lot" of children	−.10	−.36
Knowledge of reproductive physiology	.08	.69
Piped water in home	.08	.61
Primary responsibility to mother not mate	−.01	−.37
Jamaican men are irresponsible	−.01	.09
Total impregnators (age corrected)[a]	—	−.43
Total pregnancies (age corrected)[b]	—	−.41
Total visiting mates (age corrected)[c]	—	−.45

a. Below median, median, above median number for age level per pregnancy for 101 women with two or more children.

b. Below median, median, above median number for age level.

c. Below median, median, above median number for age level per 10 sexually active years.

physiology, choice of an oral contraceptive, purposeful concern with delaying the first pregnancy, and more adequate communication with the current coital partner, who is also apt to be of higher occupational status. Similarly, urban birth, too, is correlated (though less significantly than age or education) with a lower reproductive performance and with a positive attitude to contraception, choice of an oral contraceptive, and concern with delaying the first pregnancy, but not with favoring a smaller family or with more adequate communication with the sexual partner.

These independent correlations suggest that despite some changes in the availability (and perhaps acceptability) of general and sexual-reproductive education over the past generation neither the cultural matrix nor the social structure has changed sufficiently that younger respondents and other Jamaicans of similar age and socioeconomic status live, love, have sexual relations, and reproduce in a manner significantly different from the older respondents. The meaning of available contraception—and of using or not using it, competently or not—is tied less to age and generational changes than to other factors, some but not all of which are related to socioeconomic status.

Table 5 shows that education correlates with having fewer pregnancies and fewer and less varied male partners. A multiple regression analysis, however, indicates that among a variety of factors related to socioeconomic status (urban or rural birth, education, housing, mate's occupation), within a given age group only rural birth is significantly correlated with having more children, and the amount of variance thus accounted for is very small, 1.5 percent.

Thus, statistical analysis confirms what common sense suggests: sexual-reproductive behavior is a function of a whole person interacting with another, or over a lifetime with several others, in a context that encourages and reinforces or constrains and discourages certain kinds of behavior at different times in the life cycle. The separation of multiple sources of variance in this kind of behavior may obscure the meaning of life decisions, often not consciously taken, for any given person. The proportions of a population behaving in particular ways, however, and correlations between these proportions and individual social characteristics nonetheless help describe the context in which they occur.

The Personal Meaning of Age

Whatever emotional or status gain is achieved by cumulative pregnancies appears to be vitiated by the demands they place on the women locked into a more stable yet still unrewarding relationship (see chapter 8). There is a high correlation between age and wishing for fewer children: the older the woman, the unhappier she tends to be with the number of children she has produced (table 6). This correlation supports the supposition that pregnancy and childbirth are less a function of conscious, intentional management of the woman's relationship with men than of simple exposure to the possibility of sexual intercourse.

For some, increasing age means a diminution of educational and occupational aspirations. An unmarried, unemployed, 32-

Table 6. Gamma correlations of independent variables with fewer children wanted for 150 Jamaican women.

Independent variable	Fewer children wanted
Number of pregnancies, not age corrected (0-2 vs. 3-10)	.83
Number of different impregnators	.70
Total number of pregnancies, not age corrected	.69
Pregnancy (fewer, median, or more) per age	.61
Contraceptive use to delay first or space later births	− .45
Age	.45
Education	− .43
Stability of current relationship	.41
Piped water in house	− .40
Mate's occupational status	− .40
Receives financial support from mate (total/most vs. none/part)	.32
Urban birthplace (vs. town vs. rural)	− .28
Joint contraceptive decision with mate	− .24
Choice of reliable method (oral, nonoral, none)	− .23
Number of impregnators[a]	.19

a. For 101 women with two or more pregnancies.

year-old mother of five said she would like to have had more schooling and be able to read better. At this point, though, she felt she would get more from sending her children to school than from going herself.

Many expressed hope that their children "will turn out better" than they. Yet, others finally abandoned marital in favor of occupational aspirations. A 39-year-old practical nurse, the mother of four, has given up hoping for marriage: "I would prefer to better myself . . . study further, become a regular nurse."

Growing older often brings a determination to regulate fertility. Sometimes this involves deliberately downgrading the importance of sexual desire. As a 33-year-old unmarried store clerk, the mother of five, said, "I used to not want 'the control' because I was afraid it might change my nature, but now I will never get pregnant again. Having the children is something real nice, but I want to be able to care them."

On the other hand, capacity for sexual pleasure can increase when contraception is an accepted part of the conjugal relationship. One woman in her forties reported that, following an early initiation, she had disliked sexual intercourse for years. Now, four years past her last pregnancy, with a new, third, mate who wanted her to use "the planning": "*I* can have it for fun, not to make a baby."

Old age was a specific concern for many: "Children are a great comfort to you and help you when you become old." But as one said, although she would like to "count on" her children, "you can't never be sure. Them might go to England or America. If you have a boy, he get woman of his own. If you have a girl, you might care her children while she someplace else." The reliability of children as a source of old-age security seems uncertain. Most informants report this to be less true for rural areas but changing with migratory job hunting, often to the U.S., Canada, or the U.K. It is even less certain in the changing urban slum.

Born in the Country and Living in the City

The major external migratory flow from Jamaica has been to the United States, Canada, and England. Of the citizens counted in the 1970 census, only 1.88 percent had been born abroad and some of these had emigrant Jamaican parents. Emigration may have deprived Jamaica of some of its more adventurous and competent inhabitants: recent data (JIS, 1972a) show that more than half the emigrants were from the country's tiny educated class. Approximately 17 percent were professional or managerial, and 40 percent clerical or skilled. The remaining 43 percent, semi- or unskilled workers, include the majority of the women who serve as domestic help, cleaning women, and waitresses in Toronto, Washington-Baltimore, Philadelphia, and New York. In 1979-1980 Jamaican correspondents and the public news media reported an accelerated outflow of middle-class Jamaicans because of political tensions in the country.

On the island itself, internal migration seems constant. Almost 60 percent of the women with whom we spoke, including the majority of the older ones, had been born and raised on small farms or in rural cabins with garden patches. Another 21 percent came from small towns; only 19 percent had been born in metropolitan Kingston. Most still said they found Kingston "more interesting" than their native parishes. Unlike their compatriots who have remained in the country, they have had the initiative and energy to leave their homes and families and cope with a sometimes solitary existence in a new environment. This phenomenon accords with data from many other countries (Brody, 1970). Most came to the city in search of work, and some to go to school. Some also used the move to sever oppressive relationships. Several noted that they "gave up religion," symbolizing parental strictness, when they moved to the city. Others wanted to get away from harsh parents or grandparents. Nevertheless, they usually maintain viable relationships with country relatives, exchange visits, and cope with job loss or other difficulty by retreating temporarily to work or board in the rural area.

Rural origins were most frequent for Manley nonusers of contraceptives. This fits the finding of least contraception in the least industrialized and touristic parishes (Sinclair, 1974) and of higher fertility in the more remote parts of the island (Eyre, 1972a). The proportion of women of rural birth increases from 50 percent among current JFPA clients, to 55 percent among current nonusers seen at Manley, to 76.7 percent for Manley never-users. Kingston birth is correlated with a positive attitude toward contraception (gamma .42) and an attempt to have used it to delay initial or space later pregnancies (gamma .47).

Women born in the country spoke more negatively about contraception. As one who came from Westmoreland at age 18 said, "In the country after you finish school you start right in having babies." Almost 84 percent of ever pregnant respondents were of rural origin.

After the first pregnancy, however (and greater temporal distance from one's origins), reproductive performance *in relation to others of the same age group* is not related to rural or urban birth. With increasing length of urban residence, factors other than place of origin become important in determining a woman's pregnancy status in terms of her age group.

Respondents born in Kingston, in contrast with the others, tend to be younger (gamma .27), educated past primary school (gamma .39), to live in homes with piped water (gamma .63), and to have mates of higher occupational status—mainly in skilled manual jobs (gamma .29). People coming into town from the country have fewer socioeconomic assets than those of city birth and tend not to overcome their initial deficits.

An urban-rural difference in developmental experience is suggested by the tendency, independent of age, for town-reared respondents to recall their worst childhood memories in terms of emotional deprivation (gamma .34) rather than flogging. Among those of rural birth, working in the fields was often mentioned as particularly strenuous and unpleasant. The differences, however, are less impressive than the similarities: more than three-fourths of all respondents, urban and rural, characterized their childhood discipline as harsh and repressive.

Education

The degree to which lack of education reflects social circumstances or innate lack of competence is uncertain. As one young woman said, "I left after the third year because I never got much from school." Most respondents reported that their parents or guardians placed a high value on education. They also told, however, of lack of privacy and poor light, the distractions of a noisy, thickly populated dwelling, and the continuing expectation that house or garden chores would be completed before departure for school. School, even in the urban area, was often some distance from home, so that tardiness and fatigue after a long walk were frequent. As one said, "I had to help with the meals, go down and buy the milk, bring it home, and try to get to school by nine. After school over at four, rush home, wash the dishes, put up the fowls, carry water—the water pipe was about a chain [about two-thirds of a mile] away."

Another typical story illustrates the interrelationship of poverty and little education: "After father died my mother tried to support us alone. We had a few goats, a little coffee . . . were poor. I worked in the field and helped take care of the younger children, so I didn't go to school much. But now I would like to try to better myself."

In addition, there was often a sense of the teacher, usually a young woman with little education herself, representing discipline and concern with trivia rather than a sure sense of knowledge and a wish to transmit it. The teacher's lack of concern about absences was remembered: "If I missed she think I needed at home."

Within the narrow range of this working-class population, the small number of women who grew up in an environment encouraging education past primary school felt more favorable about regulating their own fertility and acting upon that feeling. Those who contracepted in order to delay their first pregnancy or space later births tended to adhere less frequently to traditional matricentric beliefs, to have had first intercourse at a later age, and more frequently to agree with their mate about contraceptive use. Because they had managed their own fertility they less often wished they had produced fewer children (table 6). They were also the least constrained by the idea that it is natural to have a foreordained number of children to be reared with the help of female relatives, and by a sense of their mates as dominant and at any event unreachable.

Those who had entered secondary school had had fewer sexual partners and fewer pregnancies than others of the same age. They tended to have received sex information from their mothers and not to hold traditional fertility-related beliefs or to believe that a woman's primary responsibility is to her mother rather than to her mate (table 5). These factors, however, are not totally dependent on education. Correlations of high reproductive performance and partner diversity with traditional beliefs remain positive; and poor partner communication and low age of initial sexual experiences remain correlated with having many pregnancies *even for the 114 women who had no more than a primary education* (table 7).

Occupation

Money and opportunities to acquire it were constant concerns. Most of our respondents could not count on the secure support of others. Underlying feelings of oppression and resentment were pervasive. Most said that for most of their lives they had worked harder than they wished. Almost none were satisfied with their jobs. All cherished some dream of self-improvement. One said she was picking up letters "for the richest people" in her district at the age of seven. By age 14 she was recording her grandmother's milk sales. At 19, after her mother had moved to the United States, she did housework for a maternal aunt. At the time of the interview, now in her mid-thirties, she was clerking in a cheap department store but would have liked to study to become a hospital dietician. Or she might have liked to "go to America," as her mother did. Unlike her mother, though, she would "earn money to send back" to bring her children over. She verbalized her resentment at being abandoned, but did not express strong feeling about it.

Another woman in her mid-thirties, a self-employed beautician, said she went to beauty school because she failed the local examinations to go on to secondary school. Now she wished she

Table 7. Gamma correlations of beliefs and sexual-reproductive behavior with fertility-related factors for 114 Jamaican women with a primary education or less. (Figures in parentheses are correlations for the entire group of 150, including those with some secondary education; no belief or behavior is included that does not have at least one probably significant correlation—gamma .30 or more—with a fertility-related factor.)

Beliefs and behaviors	Number of pregnancies for age group	Number of impregnators (women with 2 or more children)	Number of visiting mates per 10 sexually active years
Traditional beliefs			
Belief in traditional grandmother	.51 (.62)	.40 (.40)	.15 (.23)
Belief in "lot" of children	.32 (.44)	.15 (.31)	.12 (.27)
Contraceptive sexual-reproductive behavior			
Age at first pregnancy	−.51 (−.57)	−.33 (−.35)	−.31 (−.35)
Contracepted to delay first or space later pregnancies	−.43 (−.55)	−.20 (−.34)	−.26 (−.38)
Made joint contraceptive decision with current mate	−.39 (−.33)	−.50 (−.50)	−.21 (−.24)
Age at first union	−.31 (−.47)	−.21 (−.48)	−.23 (−.30)
Received sex information from mother	−.21 (−.31)	−.31 (−.38)	−.10 (−.17)
Discussed contraception with mate	−.12 (−)	−.34 (−.41)	−.37 (−.40)
Positive communication with first coital partner	−.01 (−)	−.39 (−.43)	−.23 (−.29)

had tried again and become a nurse. She felt that women can do "anything they want as long as is working."

A primary school teacher in her twenties said she was sometimes bothered by the fact that she is more intelligent than her husband. She would have liked him to go back to school. She herself wanted to go into politics and run for parliament.

A young woman whose common-law boy friend was a short-order cook had to stay home and look after her three children. She was angry because he rarely took her out and did not give her enough money, but was afraid to leave him "because life may be worse than now." She earned a little as a dressmaker at home, but could not do much because of the demands of child care. If she could have done what she wanted she would now be a secretary. She would like her children to be "the best . . . maybe a nurse or a teacher." Jamaican women, she said, "have it hard . . . No job, and if job, little pay."

A third-grade-educated, 28-year-old mother of six by three men did not have a job because she had to look after her children. The father of the last two occasionally gave her money, but "the first four will get no help." When he came to town every two weeks they slept together. She was not sure she enjoyed sexual intercourse, but said, "When you lonely it better to feel someone there." The man would have liked her "to give" him another baby, but she used a diaphragm because she "wants no more children . . . Women get more of a fair deal with this 'control.' " If she could have started over she would have liked to be a nurse and help others. Women should be able to do what they want, "be politicians or doctors or truckdrivers."

Church Attendance

Other observers have described the roots of Jamaican religious belief in Africa, the British Isles, and the United States. Olive Lewin, for example, believes that religious attitudes derived from Africa underlie many practices today. Christian beliefs "at deep levels still puzzle many Jamaicans," for whom an "instinctive view of Life, Death, and Creation makes it difficult . . . to accept a religion that seems to be focused on a particular place and a particular time. For the traditional Jamaican there is hardly any line of demarcation between what is sacred and what is secular . . . Problems that exist in the world of matter originated in some spiritual short-coming and must, therefore, be solved at a spiritual level . . . Whether the problem be legal, social or physical, it is the religious cult leader who is first consulted" (Lewin, 1974, p. 7).

The non-African roots of Jamaican religious systems include Moravian missionaries active on the island as early as 1754. Wesleyan Methodists, Baptists, and "free Negro preachers" came from the United States in the 1780s (Seaga, 1969). In the late 1850s evangelical movements in the United States, Ireland, and Great Britain arrived with the Great Revival. After reaching a peak in 1861-1862 the congregations began to dwindle away, but other short-lived movements with political and economic appeal followed. In 1920, for example, Alexander Bedward, who had previously spoken of the unsatisfactory nature of the white-dominated world, prophesied that he and his disciples of African ancestry would ascend to heaven, returning to build a new earth after the old one had been destroyed.

Revivalism still characterizes a variety of cults that share the feature of spirit possession but differ in details of dancing, singing, and particular spiritist concerns. The light-skinned, educated, and urbanized people of higher social status tend to belong to established Christian churches. The darker, less educated, country dwellers tend to belong to more pentecostal groups, where "the spirit" is more acceptable and baptism and similar rituals, including "clapping," are more prominent. Although the prevalence of actual participation in the remaining revival cults is uncertain, their influence in the healing context seems strong.

Approximately four-fifths of the women claimed membership in conventional churches. About one-fourth of these are fundamentalist or evangelical, and 12 percent each Catholic or Anglican. More than one-third of those claiming membership, however, never attended, and approximately one-fourth did so less than once a month. Many noted the intense and oppressive religiosity of parents or grandparents who were staunch members of village churches; these respondents stopped going when they left home and were no longer required to do so.

With rare exceptions the 150 respondents denied organized religion as significant for their fertility-related behavior. There are no correlations between church affiliation or attendance and reproductive performance, and most who did identify with a church said it had no specific significance in respect to sex or childbearing. A few respondents, however, refrained from using contraceptives on the grounds of evangelical, fundamentalist, or quasi-religious folk healing beliefs. Several revealed the intense personal meaning of religion in this regard. A few quoted biblical injunctions: "The Bible say blessed them the women who brings forth a child. If not you are a barren woman . . . if you don't have a child you might as well not be alive." One combined this view with concern for old age: "How will you manage when you get older if you have no children? The Lord would say, in your days of living what were you doing? You dashed your pickney away."

Some women recognized but did not act on religious attitudes concerning chastity and abortion: "When I got pregnant first and didn't want it some people said I should get an abortion. It was against my Catholic religion, but the real reason I didn't get it was that I wanted to keep the child because I didn't know if I would ever get married. I knew I would have the child."

A few spoke of religion as a general helping force in their lives. A Catholic who had not attended mass for two years wrote regularly to Oral Roberts, who "prays for me." An intense chest pain was "cured" when she went to sleep with one of his pamphlets on her bosom. Another, who in her late twenties had had four children by three men, was an Anglican who attended church every Sunday. She described herself as "very religious," and for a time attended a pentecostal church: "But it doesn't make a difference. We all worship the same God. Just one church claps and the other doesn't." Another Anglican, "born into it," had attended the Church of God since moving to Kingston and had had "the spirit descend into" her. With only minimal support from her current boy friend and concerned about the welfare of her several children, she said that prayer "helps a lot . . . Maybe it would be worse without it, and when the spirit comes down it makes me feel younger . . . happy."

Membership in a traditional church combined with regular attendance at one offering immediate spiritual contact—a widespread pattern in officially Catholic Brazil—was not uncommon. One woman, for example, went to Catholic mass each week and also to the Church of the New Testament, where "they clap." The second, she said, was "more important to me because I pray for health and to be happy." But even the traditional churches could provide a response to supplication. One woman, married, a secondary school graduate with three children, was "a traditional

Baptist—no clapping." She attended church twice monthly, believed in God, and prayed: "If you pray for something you want, after a while it works out. Most of my decisions are made by prayer." Her attitude toward reproduction, including abortion, was matter-of-fact; "If you make up your mind to do it—okay."

Some would have liked to attend church but were resigned to not going, and with the passage of time seemed to be losing interest. One young woman said, "I haven't been to mass for three years because I have to stay home with my children. I feel miserable about staying with them all the time. I thought of having an abortion with the last one . . . but it is a sin . . . but now I wonder. Maybe would have been better."

Male Respondents

We were able to collect data on 283 male JFPA clients. All but four, there to accompany their mates, came to the East Street clinic to obtain condoms for their own use. Ninety-three percent had visited at least once before, and almost three-fourths had come every few weeks for several months. Condoms are an important adjunct to their sex lives; two-thirds reported that they had intercourse three to four times weekly (table 8). Prior to coming to East Street 60 percent had obtained their supplies from drugstores and 17 percent from other family planning centers. Despite their concern with contraception, however, more than three-quarters (including 36 percent with three or more) had had children by the time of the interview.

These men were more self-confident than the women who come to the East Street clinic. Better dressed and better educated, they were at ease with the staff and often jovial with the dignified, gray-haired man who interviewed them for the project. They were friendly and seemingly open with me, too. The younger ones indulged in occasional male bragging, saying they wanted condoms for an anticipated "busy weekend." It is probable that the condoms were not all to be used with their primary partners. Some of the older ones engaged me in the commonality of our middle-aged status. They were serious, speaking with concern about

Table 8. Frequency of intercourse per week for 283 male JFPA clients.

Frequency per week	Usual (%)	In week prior to interview (%)
0	1.8	1.1
1	1.8	6.4
2	20.1	20.5
3	34.3	28.3
4	36.4	33.2
5	3.2	8.1
6	0.4	0.4
7	0.0	0.0
8	0.0	0.0
9	2.1	2.1

Note: Asked whether frequency varies with income and work or study demand, 23.3 percent said it did, 38.9 percent denied it, and 37.8 percent did not know. Asked about abstinence, 27.2 percent acknowledged frequent prolonged periods, 13.1 percent occasional abstinence, and 59.7 percent denied any. Only 3.9 percent admitted that their regular partner was not always available for intercourse.

Jamaica's population problem or about "irresponsible" young men who father babies and then don't support them. Some indicated they had younger sexual partners "on the side." One wanted to talk with me about his problem in "getting a stand." But concern about erectile potency was rarely expressed.

The Meaning of Age in Contraceptive Use

The youngest male who came for condoms was 15; the two oldest, 53 and 57. Eighty-six percent were between ages 21 and 42. The predominance of young adults may reflect a variety of factors, from intensity of sexual desire to the primary partner's age, through attitudes toward birth limitation. Only a few indicated that the condoms were for disease prevention. One of the older men mentioned that his common-law wife no longer "saw her period" and that he needed his "French letters" because he didn't want "to give a baby" to a younger, visiting partner.

Older men, like the women, tended to be less urban in origin and less educated than the younger respondents. They also had less educated mates with whom most, by then, were cohabiting and felt they knew well. Optimism about the future of the current relationship, however, was only weakly correlated with age. As with the female respondents, the persistence of a partnership did not engender a feeling of security about its future.

Older men predictably preferred larger families and reproductively compliant women. Relatively few had contracepted prior to fathering their first child and, as with the women, age is correlated with having produced more children. Unlike older women with many children, though, age for these men does not correlate with a wish for fewer children (table 9). They see the man as the central figure in a heterosexual relationship; the woman's needs

Table 9. Significant and insignificant gamma correlations of status, beliefs, and behavior with age for 283 Jamaican men.

Factors	Age
Significant	
Education	− .36
Urban birth	− .32
Feels knows primary mate well	.41
Primary mate's education	− .32
Cohabiting status	.47
Number of children	.64
Larger ideal family size	.66
Optimistic about future of current relationship	.24
A woman should risk pregnancy to gain a husband	.30
Story heroine agrees to man's request to have a baby for him	.35
Used effective contraception prior to fathering first child	− .60
Insignificant	
Occupation	− .09
Wants fewer children	.03
Church attendance	− .01
Age of first coitus	.05
Understanding of reproductive physiology	− .13
Joint contraceptive decision with mate	.05
Frequency of intercourse	.07
Pregnancy is uncontrollable	.07
Favors abortion	− .10
Story heroine agrees to have a white man's baby	.04
Agrees with story heroine's decision to abort	− .12

and independence are clearly viewed as subordinate. Thus, they tended more often to believe that a woman should risk pregnancy to gain a husband, and to identify a story heroine as assenting to a man's request that she have a baby for him. Nevertheless, certain behaviors associated with a more modern or liberal status are not related to age. These include church attendance, knowledge of reproductive physiology, and abstract attitudes to such matters as abortion. Nor did they appear to have had their first sexual intercourse at a significantly different age than the younger men.

Almost four-fifths acknowledged regular sexual contacts in addition to their primary partner (including visiting unions and pickups). The highest proportion of men with multiple partners, 55 percent, is between ages 25 and 34. After age 35 there is some reduction in diversity and an increase in the number of cohabiting unions, but not a reported reduction in frequency of intercourse. These men, approximately five years older than their mates' median age, had achieved sufficient economic stability to contribute something to their support. This encourages living together, which permits them to maintain their level of sexual intercourse by having a woman to sleep with every night.

Although the church attendance pattern was similar to that of the women, fewer men, as might be expected for the more economically secure, were nonaffiliated. Only 9.2 percent belonged to fundamentalist or evangelical groups. These findings also fit their more urban background: 37.8 percent, almost twice the proportion of women respondents, were Kingston born.

Social Status and Sexual-Reproductive Performance

Higher-status, urban-born respondents tended to have better educated mates. Almost half of their primary sexual partners had progressed beyond primary school. Nearly 30 percent were full-time housewives. More than half were employed in nonmanual occupations; only 16 percent worked at manual jobs. Like their mates, almost 16 percent owned land. These better educated couples, however, did not have stable cohabiting relationships. Rather, it is the lower-status (gamma .57), more rural (gamma .48) partners who tended to be currently cohabiting, and the cohabiters had more children than other men in their age group (gamma .48). Higher-status men, compared with others their age, tended on the contrary to have visiting mates (gamma .32) and fewer children (gamma .26). Thus, within this group of contraceptive users sexual partnerships were less institutionalized than those of lower-status men of comparable age. They seemed unready to settle down, and had no apparent interest in signifying their unions by having their mate produce a child "for" them. In addition, they more often approved of independent behavior in women, expressing positive attitudes toward abortion and to story heroines who consider abortion for unwanted pregnancy and do not submit to a man's pressure to have a baby for him. They were negative about a woman's risking pregnancy in order to gain marriage, and were not so disturbed as lower-class men about female sterility (table 10).

Similarly, the higher-status men within the group knew more about reproductive physiology, had more often used effective contraception prior to their first child, and were less inclined than those of lower status to want a large family. It is clear that at this stage of their lives they were interested in being able to enjoy sexual intercourse without reproducing. Nevertheless, they were no more inclined than the lower-status men to negotiate contraceptive use with their mates (except to suggest that the latter continue to use their own methods as well); fertility control for them appears primarily to be a private effort. They did not share contraceptive responsibility, but managed it themselves in order to maintain their freedom from additional family and conjugal ties, perhaps as they pursued their careers. Accordingly, they more often acknowledged having abstinent periods and tended not to have fathered babies with several women. For them personal mobility and freedom to have sexual pleasure appeared to be more important as a means of personal affirmation and self-esteem than did reproductive prowess and a public image of unrelenting, sexually aggressive masculinity.

In sharp contrast to the female respondents, almost half the fathers in this sample had contracepted effectively before having

Table 10. Gamma correlations of fertility-related factors with socioeconomic factors for 283 male JFPA clients.

Fertility-related factors	Education	Literacy	Piped water	Occupation	Mate's education	Urban birth
Attitudes						
Negative to female sterility	−.34	−.79	−.47	−.26	−.34	.17
Larger ideal family size	−.29	.03	−.12	−.11	−.29	−.26
Story heroine submits to man's wish for baby	−.34	−.28	−.27	−.31	−.39	−.14
Story heroine considers abortion	.28	.53	.17	.23	.21	.09
A woman should risk pregnancy for marriage	−.63	−.76	−.82	−.47	−.62	−.37
Favors abortion	.44	.83	.48	.32	.42	.00
Favors mate's contracepting	−.02	.13	−.04	.07	.06	−.03
Contraceptive behavior						
Effective contraception prior to first child	.65	.40	.58	.40	.58	.39
Use of male and female methods for reliability	.17	.18	.26	.26	.15	.06
Communication with partner						
Feels knows mate well	−.01	.19	.38	.01	.06	−.03
Optimistic about future of primary relationship	−.04	.35	.43	.05	.17	−.18
Discussed contraception with mate	−.28	−.10	−.18	−.22	−.06	−.12
Made joint contraceptive decision	.09	−.06	.12	.15	.13	.11
Sexual history						
Age at first coitus	.02	−.06	.08	−.01	.12	.04
Coital frequency per week	−.09	−.03	−.05	−.12	−.07	.00
Acknowledges periods of abstinence	.29	.13	.07	.20	.13	.12
Knowledge of reproductive physiology	.79	.81	.76	.45	.78	.05
A different woman for each of 2 children (N:161)	−.36	−.48	−.24	−.31	—	−.14

their first child. This contraceptive use is related to education, chiefly to having completed primary school (gamma .76) and to its corollaries: occupational status, urban birth, and piped water in the home. Their less traditional attitudes are reflected in their feeling that a woman should not risk pregnancy to gain a husband (gamma .59), should not accept a man's request to "have a baby for him" (gamma .52), and a small ideal family size (gamma .56). They did not, however, unequivocally favor abortion.

The men with the most children, like the women, were the oldest and least educated who began using condoms late in their reproductive careers. Among the younger and better educated men, unintended failure was often due to the unavailability of a condom or to impulsive neglect, as when intoxicated. In some instances the man said his female partner had wanted a child and made it difficult for him to use his "French letter."

More than one-third of the group (37.1 percent) wished they had fewer children and 71.4 percent, including many who were childless, did not wish more than they presently had. Those with the most children in their age group strongly wished they had fewer (gamma .57). As noted above, this wish is not related to age itself (gamma .03). All therefore used the condom with their "outside" or secondary mates and two-thirds did so with their primary mates. They reported that one-fourth of their primary mates also used a contraceptive method, mainly the pill and in a few cases a diaphragm or foam. Almost three-quarters of these women did so, according to the man, because they were unsure about the future of the relationship. Only a few men (7.9 percent) engaged in technically unprotected intercourse with their primary mates (who may no longer be menstruating), but some of these practiced withdrawal or rhythm with varying consistency.

A wish to avoid the economic burden of children was given by more than three-quarters as the main reason for contracepting with their primary mate, and with their regular outside mate for somewhat fewer. Other reasons included being too young to have a family or not wanting to be tied down. Contraceptive use had increased over time; only 62.2 percent reported having used a condom or cooperative method with a previous mate. Reasons for nonuse among the 90 percent with a previous mate were obscure, evenly divided between "none" and "insufficient motivation."

Only one-fourth of the men reported that their decision to contracept or not, or about which method to use, was reached with their partner's participation. These men felt positively about their mates' using a contraceptive and were sufficiently concerned about reliability to try to ensure it with the combined use of male and female methods. These respondents were not, however, the most educated or occupationally advanced group still in visiting unions who wished small families. On the contrary, they tended to live with partners whom they felt they knew well (gamma .42) and to be optimistic about the future of the union (gamma .29). They had larger ideal family sizes (gamma .37) and generally did not wish fewer children than they already had (gamma .27). That is, they were not preventing but spacing future births with the aim of enhancing the quality of life for themselves and the families they had already started.

Although men with more children than others their age tended to wish they had fewer, they nonetheless (perhaps reflecting an adaptation to reality) had a larger ideal family size than did men with fewer children. They did not espouse all of the more prevalent traditional rural attitudes, but were male dominant in viewpoint. A woman should risk pregnancy to gain a husband (gamma .34), and children without marriage are all right (gamma .39); in keeping with this attitude, they reported more frequent sexual intercourse (gamma .30). Age at first intercourse, however (perhaps because it is universally low), does not seem related to either coital or reproductive performance. Although these men with a high reproductive performance tend to be among those less socioeconomically advantaged, the negative association between socioeconomic status and reproductive performance is much less marked than for the female respondents.

Traditional male-dominant attitudes have sexual-reproductive corollaries independent of age and education. Even among the 140 men with no more than a primary school education, those who perceived a story heroine as assenting to a man's wish that she have a baby for him tended to have more than the median number of children for their age (gamma .29). A male-dominant attitude is similarly correlated with belief in the traditional grandmother's role (gamma .36). The prevalence of male-dominant views throughout the group of 283 suggests their cultural similarity to the less socioeconomically advantaged majority who do not contracept. Only 11 percent unreservedly favored abortion. Almost all believed strongly in the woman's primary responsibility to her mate and children, and in the father's primary economic responsibility for all. Most (84 percent) felt that Jamaican women are better off than men. Approximately three-fourths regarded sterility as a bad thing, and half thought a woman should risk pregnancy to obtain a husband and that it is all right to have children without marriage. Nevertheless, three-fourths said that single-parent families headed by the mother are bad for the children. More than twice as many regarded fatherhood, in contrast to motherhood, as requiring important knowledge, skill, and responsibility.

Reactions to story situations suggest that these men expect women to produce babies when asked to. Most identified a heroine as accepting a man's request for a baby in return for his support of her and her previous children. Very few felt that she or a woman without children would reject such an offer. A majority perceived a story heroine as carrying a pregnancy to term, not seeking abortion despite lack of support.

Socioeconomic Status and Fertility-Related Attitudes and Behavior of Men and Women

These findings fit the general pattern documented by a number of studies in different societies over several years (see, for example, Ryder, 1959; United Nations, 1953).

Better educated, economically secure men and women tended to espouse small-family values and more autonomy and self-determination for women. They tended more often to contracept in order to delay initial or space later pregnancies. The sexual-reproductive patterns associated with more advantaged social status were more prevalent among Kingston-born respondents, who were on the average younger than inmigrants from rural areas. Younger women in particular were more likely to have obtained sexual information at an early age, especially from public sources. In this respect the changing social structure may allow sexual-reproductive aims and feelings to emerge with less conflict into awareness, although not necessarily into more effective action, than in the past.

Although increasing age is associated with increasing conjugal stability, the older female respondents experienced little economic or emotional security. Despite longer-term relationships, they tended to wish they had fewer children (table 4). The better educated women with higher status mates who had used contraception successfully tended not to wish that they had fewer children. They had more options in life from an earlier age and used their knowledge and freedom to regulate their own fertility.

The more well-to-do condom-using males appear to achieve more satisfying relationships with age. Those with most children tended to be of lower socioeconomic status. They are less trapped, however, by early parenthood associated with a wish to demonstrate their fertility, symbolize status, or signify or solidify relationships by having children. They deliberately used contraceptives over which they exerted sole control in order to maintain freedom from conjugal and parental responsibilities until they were ready for them.

The Value of Children

In this society the value of children seems tied to the impact of growing up in a particular socioeconomic stratum. Developmental experience at the lowest level socializes a person into a sense of powerlessness and passive acceptance of the influences impinging on her or his life. Supplication, rather than recourse to a feared or distrusted technology, is the alternative to passivity. Contraceptive methods represent the unfamiliar and alien. Suspicion and withdrawal are easier than optimistic expectancy and approach. The seemingly symptomatic corollaries of life at the lowest socioeconomic level are adaptive as they reflect the survival demands of reality. Children become valuable as companions for old age rather than simply sources of economic support. Providing psychosocial security and a continuing familiar connection with life and the community, children embody the values of lifelong knowledge and reciprocal obligation. Parenthood is an available source of self-affirmation and self-discovery as well as status in a society with few alternative roles. Producing children is also a symbolic means of demonstrating environmental control over life—the external reality—through the achievement of inner control—the accomplishment of impregnation and delivery.

On the other hand, creating a family without the means to care for it impedes personal mobility, health, and growth. Furthermore, child production may be an instrumental rather than expressive pattern: the child itself may be exploited. To the degree that unprotected coitus and having children reduce unconscious anxiety, guilt, or other tension; afford disguised expression for unacceptable aims or wishes; increase the actual life difficulties of parents; and occur under circumstances that limit the child's life chances, they may be regarded as symptomatic acts as well as maladaptive ones. This view is made more plausible by the seemingly obligatory quality of reproductive acts that are carried out in opposition to conscious or so-called rational opinion. With few exceptions, a sample of 240 Jamaican working-class women in the 1960s (Netherlands, 1968) agreed with the statement "It is hardly fair to bring a child into the world with the way things look for the future." In the 1970s, however, despite the availability of new techniques for limiting fertility, Jamaican men and women continued to bring children into a world that they still regarded as harsh and exploitative.

6 Relationship with Mother, Menarche, and First Intercourse

If I looked at a boy, she would flog me.

When the blood came, I felt fear.

His mother was away one day so we went to his room. I didn't know what he was doing and it hurt, but later we did it again, and then I began to know what it was.

Female respondents

The outlines of collective experience as well as of unique biography emerge quickly in intimate therapeutic discourse with patients. The psychiatrist, though, lacks the ethnographer's opportunity to participate in the everyday life of the people being studied; he depends for his data on clinical interaction in an office or hospital setting. But this can sometimes be supplemented. At the end of one clinic morning at UWI there appeared a 48-year-old man who had been sitting in the courtyard. He wanted to talk, he said, about his "nervousness," but it soon developed that his real concern was with his common-law wife. Because she would not come to the hospital we arranged a visit to his "yard" in West Kingston.

The yard was a large, square, dusty space with one side separated from the narrow, unpaved street by a metal fence, itself obscured by luxuriantly flowering bushes coated with a thin film of dust. The other three sides were formed by single-storied wooden buildings, their paint dulled by neglect, façades bumpy with boards of varied size and color applied to apparent defects in the walls. Protruding into the space were several ramshackle structures sheltering cooking areas. Criss-crossing all was a maze of lines supporting a wilderness of laundry, whipping in the occasional breeze, glaring white against the bright blue, cloudless sky. People seemed to be constantly coming and going into and out of the yard and various doorways, stopping together briefly, then moving apart. Two small boys, absorbed in private play, squatted in the patch of shade provided by a banana tree in one corner.

We entered one of the doorways. In the relative gloom, together on a single couch, sat three young women smiling widely. Each held a baby to her breast. My patient introduced them as his three daughters, aged 16, 18, and 21, and pointed out the first child of the oldest girl playing on the floor nearby. Their mother, his common-law wife, was crouched mutely on a stool in the kitchen lean-to. A child, identified as her 5-year-old son by another man, stood at her knee, the fingers of one hand in his mouth, the other clutching the hem of the short skirt riding high on her thigh. Four other children were not at home.

The man was clearly proud of his healthy, plump, smiling daughters and his grandchildren; but he spoke bitterly of the "shiftless" men who had impregnated them and contributed little to their support. He thought that if her mother had not become progressively "sick in the head" for the past several years (caused, he believed, by her own last pregnancy), the 16-year-old at least would not yet have had a child. By this he meant she would have been a virgin, for he was unequivocal in his opposition to "the control," which he felt was immoral and potentially dangerous to health. The girl herself, however, did not share his unhappiness and smiled at her father as she contradicted him. I took advantage of the visit, although I was officially there for her mother, to explore the situation. Yes, "it true," she had been surprised and upset to discover herself pregnant. She had not expected it because, as she described her first intercourse, "me felt nothing but bad when him put it in me." At first she felt guilty and ashamed as well as angry at her parents for having taught her nothing about sex or reproduction. She was also lonely because her boy friend, a somewhat older man who worked intermittently in a nearby shoe repair shop, disappeared after denying paternity. She was especially disappointed because "him nice to me." She was "sick to me stomach" and "felt miserable" for about two months. Later, her boy friend reappeared and she took some pleasure in vengefully refusing his invitation to come live with him "so then him could say I had the baby for him." She considered staying with her aunt, her father's sister, but began to enjoy talking with her girlfriends about the approaching baby and preferred to stay with her sisters because "them could tell me what to do." She did not consider it unusual, upon my pointing it out, that although her sisters and aunt could tell her what to do about taking care of herself during pregnancy and could help her make arrangements for the delivery, they had not given her any useful information about sex and reproduction except to warn her that with menarche she was vulnerable to pregnancy. As she said, "You don't talk about things like that, auntie would flog—better to be quiet."

The other two girls chimed in. They too had been dismayed and upset upon becoming pregnant. "Nobody ever expect anything happen." The two older girls had been beaten violently by their mother when, fearfully, they had confessed the disappearance of their periods. She shouted that they had disgraced her, were trying to grow up too quickly, and threatened to expel them from the house. When the youngest became pregnant, the mother was already withdrawn and paid little attention, but "auntie" had spoken "crossly" with her. The father himself had been angry (at the moment of this conversation he had drifted out into the yard and was chatting with a friend), but had talked mainly about being ashamed and did not threaten them.

Each girl was happy with her first baby, but the oldest said she had not wanted the second. She had conceived in order to "have a baby for" a second boy friend, but when he went off to Canada in her fourth month of pregnancy, she had inquired both at the hospital and from friends about the possibility of abortion. The people at the hospital told her that she was too far along, and although a friend had recommended a tea made with pennyroyal she had decided that she might regret losing the baby, especially if she never had another.

None of the sisters had considered contraception, although all knew about the JFPA services. Despite their continuing sexual exposure, none felt themselves at risk of pregnancy, for they were still nursing. The oldest said she was going to East Street one day to find out more about "the planning." She would not tell her newest boyfriend, however, because "them think that with the planning you are going with other men, and them never know."

A question about abstinence as a possible way of regulating fertility provoked a storm of giggles. Finally the oldest, apparently regarded as a spokeswoman by the other two, said, referring to the men, "Them want it." The rejoinder "And how do you feel about it?" provoked another storm. The 16-year-old remained silent. The 18-year-old said she wasn't sure if she liked it but she thought it necessary "to stay healthy." The oldest said she had gotten to like it sometimes, but she really did it for her boy friend. Although she had heard that having relations and "not going against your nature" were important to health, especially of "the mind," she didn't believe it.

Later I tried to engage the mother in conversation as the man hovered nearby. Her replies to questions were monosyllabic, her most forceful responses physical as she held her son to her as a shield between us. In time her eldest daughter joined us. I learned that the woman was 38 and had been 17 at the birth of her first child. The little boy was named after the man, George, who was presumably the father. The daughter said matter-of-factly that her parents had "had a fuss" about four years ago, her father had moved temporarily into the home of a "girl friend who had already had a baby for him" and whom he still visited regularly, and George "had come looking for" her mother. About her mother she said, "She funny in the head for long time, but him George him not care." She herself had had "two babies for" two men and now had a third boy friend. She thought that next year they might rent a room where they could live together. For the moment she was content to be with him on weekends and anyway her mother needed her more. She stroked her mother's hair affectionately as she said this. In time we moved the conversation to her mother's need for hospitalization. The eldest daughter agreed to care for little George, although her father suggested that he should go to big George's mother. I left to make the necessary arrangements. Later I saw the patient on the psychiatric ward at UWI. She was visited regularly by her daughters, who came bringing little George with them. Her mate also came but remained on the periphery of the group.

Menarche and First Intercourse

Menarche, for many of our JFPA clients and Manley patients, was the disturbing discovery of "blood." It occurred for four-fifths of the 150 respondents between the ages of 12 and 15, with a median of 14. Once the new status of menstruating woman is established the next step toward social maturity is anticipated. This is sexual intercourse. The earliest age of reported first inter-course was 9, the oldest 25. Most (87.3 percent), though, re-ported a first experience between the ages of 14 and 19, with a median of 17 years. This median is identical with Blake's report of almost 20 years earlier (Blake, 1961). However, the 133 ever pregnant of the 150 respondents had a mean age of first inter-course of 15.3 years, suggesting a possible drop in the age of first heterosexual exploration.

Almost two-thirds of the 150 had had intercourse within four years after starting to menstruate; the correlation between age at menarche and that at first intercourse is positive though weak (gamma .27). Respondents who had first intercourse in the same year as menarche or earlier were those who began to menstruate at a somewhat later age—14 to 18, with one at age 13. Those who began a year or more after menarche were from age 10 to 18 when they began to menstruate. It seems probable that girls whose menses do not appear when expected, at approximately the same age as their friends and sisters, eventually feel pressed to have intercourse without waiting. There was no significant correlation between age at first intercourse or other aspects of sex and menarche noted below and the age of the respondent. Rather, initial sexual behavior appears to reflect shared values and attitudes that have not changed significantly with the advent of new reproductive technologies.

The motivation for having intercourse the first time was usually difficult for the woman to formulate in retrospect. The most frequent reason, given by 38 percent, was curiosity, often linked with having menstruated for some time. As one woman said, "I felt it was time for me to have the experience," and another, "I thought I ought to get to know what it was like to be a woman." Another 25 percent said they acceded to their partner's request because they "liked" or "loved" him.

The most striking aspect of first coitus is its immediacy, the lack of a period of preliminary experience with the tender, romantic, or more diffuse caressing aspects of sex. For almost one-third the initial sexual contact was the act of intercourse itself. Although it was often preceded by their partner's exploration of their body, this is usually remembered as brief or localized: "Him felt me and the next I knew he was trying to push it in." With few exceptions previous masturbation was denied and the vulva and vagina were treated as though they were silent or anesthetic areas: "Me not know he was doing it until it pained." The sexual act itself was also brief, mainly because of the male partner's rapid ejaculation: "We got on the bed while mother was out. Him put his hand in me panties and pulled down. When he touched me there it felt funny and me not know what to do. Then came a noise outside, tried to push him away, said, 'No, not now,' but him kept on and into me. I knew then it came out of him—you know, the come—and then he let me up." For most of the others a period of petting or caressing, long enough to be remembered as such, was also soon followed by intercourse.

It is clear that these women did not learn adult sexual behavior in a manner that permitted exploration of sensual or interpersonal nuances; the act of copulation, for them, cannot be equated with complete sexual experience. Almost 17 percent said they were "forced," and careful examination of their stories suggests that at least 5 of 25 making this statement were in fact raped by older men. For others it seems likely that, having helped arrange the circumstances of a private meeting or having progressed to the point of close physical contact, they suddenly felt the need to escape or became anxious about an occurrence they had not adequately understood or predicted.

The "forced" statement, and "chance" or "no reason" for first coitus given by another one-fifth may also reflect retrospective denial or abdication of responsibility for the event. This possibility is suggested by the frequency with which they reported that they were nonetheless glad it had happened or that it had strengthened their relationship with their boy friend. This last, reported by 70 percent, may contain an element of rationalization. It can also suggest that, despite private emotional turbulence and ambivalence about the experience, it was for a majority a positive symbolic event enhancing both their private and public statuses as socially and sexually desirable females and as members of a couple. Nevertheless, although the first partner for 70 percent of the respondents was sufficiently familiar to be characterized as a "boy friend," affectional ties were cited by only one-fourth as the reason for intercourse.

The first coital partner was younger than the respondent in only one instance, the same age in 16 cases, and older in every other case. While the majority were between 1 and 6 years older, two were more than 20 years the girl's senior and both of these had probably committed rape; the five probable rapists were all at least 11 years older than the respondents. Although no probable rapist was identified as a relative, two were "boarders" in the home and one was the mother's "boy friend." Another was a "friend of the family."

Feelings About Menarche and First Intercourse

Only a few of the respondents (7.3 percent) reacted positively to the discovery that they were menstruating for the first time or anticipated the idea of becoming an adult woman as something good or positive (8.7 percent). Most (68.7 percent) were ashamed, disgusted, frightened, or ill. They experienced the event as an unwanted, usually unexpected, and not totally explicable appearance of blood from a place they had learned to ignore or regard as bad. As one said, she was "too worried to tell anyone, because I didn't know it was something like that." Another: "When I saw the blood on me panty I felt it danger." And another: "I thought a part of my body had burst out . . . afraid to tell my mother she flog me." And another: "I felt that something bad had happened inside me, something gone wrong. My sister had told me earlier, but I didn't think it had to happen to everybody."

Even those who felt close to their mothers were upset: "I was 16 when I began to see my period. I telephoned her at work and began crying, mummy come quick, something is wrong, terrible . . . After, even when I knew, I felt so crawly, everything that was bad, would it show . . . I was so ashamed." Many felt so strongly that they had undergone something dirty, disgusting, or "bad" that they waited a day or two before telling an older woman about it.

A final 24 percent of the women expressed themselves in relatively flat terms as having been and still remaining indifferent or neutral to the event. They remembered it, but "it no different me." Or "It come, nothing to do about." Or "It just the blood. What to say?" These tend to be women who have not communicated well with their mates (gamma .37), are nonliterate (gamma .32), and regard grandmothers highly (gamma .31). There are no significant generational differences between the respondents in this respect (age, gamma $-.14$).

For more than half the respondents, the idea of entering adult female status, symbolized by menarche with its sexual and reproductive connotations, evoked fear, worry, or pessimism. Almost as many, 41.3 percent, said they were indifferent or neutral about "becoming a grown-up woman." This high figure may reflect the fact that many, at the time of the interview, were disillusioned with the conditions of adult life.

Although first intercourse was desired and anticipated by most, almost half reported the actual experience as negative, painful, or disgusting. The central problem was less the accompanying physical pain than lack of positive, mutually expressive communication with the first partner. Only 59 percent reported meaningful or supportive communication. The rest stated that communication was so minimal as to be meaningless or absolutely nonexistent. Only about one-third of the women remember it positively as either pleasurable or exciting.

Individual descriptions vary widely. For example, "I didn't understand the facts of life, even though I was 20 years old, because my grandfather was a Christian and nobody told me. One night a boy I had seen on the street before asked me to a show and my aunt said I could go. After, we went to his mother's house —she was out working, and we went to his room. I didn't know what he did to me but I didn't like it, I felt sick. Later my passage began burning me, it got all swollen. We did it later, maybe about once a month because he was working in other towns. After about a year I got to enjoy it a little more."

Another woman also had her first experience at age 20 although "I had the impulse from 14." He was a student. "It was his idea. I knew nothing about it. He used a condom. I didn't enjoy it. It hurt. I really did it to please him, so I didn't feel disappointed. I didn't tell him how it felt because I was afraid he would leave me. We broke up after two years because I heard he had another girl. I never did get to like it until this year [age 27] when I went to the priest with my present boy friend and we decided to get married. I felt secure."

A more casual account of first coitus at age 16: "It was with a school friend. We were doing lessons together, then one day his mother was away. I was afraid and wished I didn't have to do it. Then we did it three more times in that month. I still hadn't made my mind up . . . was trying to learn about it . . . Then I didn't see my period." Occasionally the girl planned it. One respondent at age 17 "just wanted to get pregnant. It was somebody I knew a long time. We rented a room in a private house. It was painful but later I came to enjoy it. I knew I could have a baby and wanted one. When I told my mother she didn't say anything."

Twenty-two women, not distinguishable as a group by age or socioeconomic characteristics, described themselves as having been indifferent to or neutral about their first experience of inter-course. These tended to express the traditional view of a Ja-maican woman's role: she is important as the mother of the next generation. The single highest positive correlation with this retro-spective indifference (gamma .60) is the idea that grandmothers have crucial roles in homemaking and child rearing. (A weaker but positive correlation, .27, was present between interview flat-ness in general and having been reared by a grandmother.) They also believed it is desirable for a woman to have a baby at any cost, with or without a consistent, supportive male partner (gamma .35). In other words, they did not regard marriage, legal or common-law, as important for the security or happiness of the young woman, pregnant or a mother, or of her child. Not surpris-ingly, these 22 women tended not to report good communication or satisfaction with their current mates (gamma .40). Restated, those who reported an indifferent response to initial intercourse placed primary value on their affective bonds with older female relatives. In contrast, they were relatively unsatisfied with and had few expectations from their male partners, with whom, as a rule, they had discussed neither sex nor contraception.

The Family Context of Development

The most significant relationship influencing a girl's feelings and attitudes about becoming an adult woman is that with her mother or the person who took her mother's place. Almost two-thirds (62.7 percent) of the women (regardless of age or socioeconomic status at the time of interview) grew up in homes with their own mother present most of the time before they were 15 years old. About the same proportion (68 percent) regarded themselves as having "been reared" by their mother or a surrogate. When the mother is at home the father, but not the grandmother, tends to be there as well. Households with several maternal generations, some more aptly characterized as a female band, are not orga-nized around a consistently present mother. The alternative is one headed by a clearly dominant isolated mother, sometimes with a relative or friend to help with child care.

Fifty-six women, more than one-third of the sample, reported having been reared by someone other than their mother. In 12 instances the mother had died. In 11 she had emigrated, leaving the child behind. In the rest of the cases the respondent's mother had "passed me on" to someone else to rear. While this was often said in a matter-of-fact way it was invariably possible, with the women with whom I spoke personally, to infer if not to elicit feelings of anger or abandonment.

Women reared by their own mothers tended to have more self-esteem and feelings of self-worth, indicated by higher occupational aspirations than among those without a consistently present mother. They tended to be older at the time of first coitus and to have had a more positive first experience (figure 1). Perhaps in consequence of these circumstances they also tended to be in more stable current unions, indicated by their more often receiving financial support from their mates.

Women without mothers looked to grandmothers, friends, older female neighbors, and occasionally teachers for help and advice at menarche. Very few turned to their father at this time. One who was "ashamed and confused" at menarche said, "My mother died when I was small and father was not able to explain things to me." Another, left with a cousin after her mother's death when she was 11: "I had feelings when the blood came . . . but I was not properly looked after." This respondent could not recall details of her initial coital experience.

Fewer than half the respondents (47.3 percent) reported that their natural father was present in the home most of the time before they were 15. Only six (4 percent) described themselves as having been reared primarily by father or a surrogate. The close availability of a male parent during this important developmental period is negatively correlated with attitudes regarding mother and grandmother (gamma −.37) as the necessary center of attention; grandmothers were not significant figures in most homes in which the natural father was present (gamma −.74). These women were also negative about unmarried motherhood (gamma .29) and tended to regard men as irresponsible (gamma .34). This may be a consequence of their father's distrust of other men and

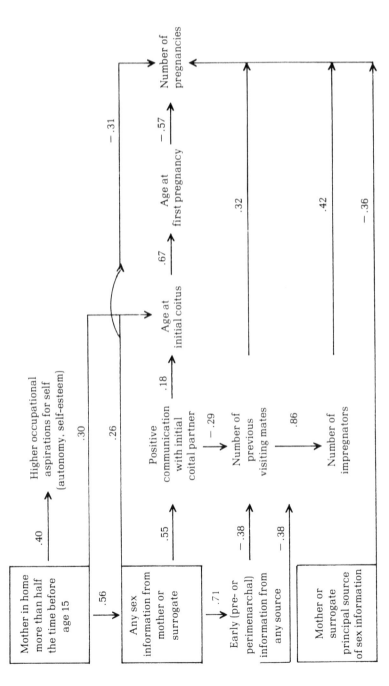

Figure 1. Maternal relationship and initial coitus in the fertility behavior sequence of 150 Jamaican women (correlative index, gamma).

the girl's feeling (in contrast with the matricentric view) that her life will depend to some degree upon men, who must therefore be regarded with caution. The variable quality of the paternal relationship and its protective and modeling importance are suggested by the positive though statistically insignificant correlations between the presence of a father and indexes of the respondent's relationships with her male partners. Those include emotional satisfaction with her current mate, having discussed contraception with him, and greater duration of the first sexual union. The presence of the natural father was not significantly correlated with indexes of socioeconomic status.

Only one-fourth of the women (26.7 percent) stated that a grandmother was in the home most of the time, and 17.3 percent were reared by a grandmother. These were mainly broken homes rather than those with extended families, so women reared in these settings present correlations contrasting with those for homes in which mother or father was present. They were matricentric, relatively unsuspicious of men (gamma .35)—perhaps because they did not expect to depend upon them—and felt positive about unmarried motherhood (gamma .52). Fewer had high occupational aspirations for themselves (gamma −.27) or their daughters (gamma −.31). Perhaps in keeping with their low ambitions, they tended to have had more visiting mates according to age (gamma .33) and impregnators per pregnancy (gamma .28) than women benefiting from direct parental guidance. This, too, may be associated with resignation or tolerance for male lack of responsibility. Such tolerance may also reflect lack of instruction by a protective paternal guardian who views other men as dangerous to his own females. Women reared in these grandmother-dominated households tended to be flat (not affectively responsive) (gamma .27) or emotionally tense (gamma .25) during interviews, suggesting less poise and interpersonal competence.

Early Memories

A general evaluation of childhood as happy characterizes almost three-fourths of the respondents. Some contrasted their childhood memories with their present status: "My children now don't have that happy time." The women most likely to look back on childhood as happy had received sex information from their mothers or a surrogate (gamma .76). This knowledge had also been acquired early enough—about the time of menarche (gamma .43)—to give them both an awareness of the reproductive meaning of sexual intercourse and enough personal security to understand intercourse as a mutual act rather than one imposed upon them. They tended to recall positive communication with their first coital partner (gamma .39) and, in contrast to uninformed women without mothers, felt negative about unmarried motherhood (gamma .36). Marriage or sharing a dwelling with a man was for them a more valued state than it was for those with the neutral or unhappy memories often associated with a less stable context of development. These last, who tended not to have had an open, communicative, and reciprocally affective relationship with their mother, also tended not to have communicated positively with their first coital partner, and to prefer unmarried to married motherhood. There were many exceptions, however. Thus, one recalled childhood as unhappy because her father "had children with other woman," but her mother "kept the balance." In this instance, it was her father who was "strict" and would not let her "go to parties."

More than half the women regarded "flogging" and more than one-fourth (28 percent) emotional loss or deprivation as their worst early memory. For the former, a beating with belt, cord, or broomstick, or simply an open-handed cuffing was inflicted as often as daily or as rarely as once or twice a week. Reasons given range from not coming straight home from school to "staying out late," "going out," "looking at boys," being "cheeky and rude," "not studying," or simple disobedience.

Memories of childhood deprivation include poverty, punishment, and the deaths of important people. Those recalling such deprivation seem more rigid and self-aware, perhaps conscientious, in their behavior, while those recalling flogging are less so. Recalling deprivation is correlated with a closer relationship with mother, higher socioeconomic status, and urban origins; it fits the relationship found in many societies between these features and depressed behavior (Brody, 1973). The women—often more privileged and of urban birth—who recalled emotional loss or deprivation as "worst" memories were less likely to have had many impregnators or to resent parents for failure to inform them, and were characterized more by contraceptive persistence and purposefulness, agreement with their mates about contracepting, and greater interest in female autonomy (attributing to a story heroine a favorable attitude toward abortion). In contrast, those—often less privileged and of rural upbringing—who recalled being flogged as their "worst" memory tended to have had more sexual partners and to be more resentful of parents. The degree to which these correlations are a consequence of the actual experience of being deprived or beaten—of living in the privileged or disadvantaged contexts characterized by these forms of punishment—or reflect antecedent psychological characteristics that led a woman to recall either emotional deprivation or flogging as her worst memory, remains uncertain.

Almost one-third of the sample denied the presence of any early memories at all. Upon request and repeated gentle probing they could say only that their earliest years (usually referring to preschool, but with the upper limit ranging as high as age ten) were simply blank. Aside from a general impression of happiness or sadness they could produce nothing specific. Adhering to traditional female and folk viewpoints, such as believing in a predestined "lot" of children (gamma .52), opposed to abortion, and passive in many respects (including acquiescence to having a baby in return for male support), more of these nonremembering women reported early first coitus (gamma .34) and conjugal unions (gamma .31). Of special interest as an indicator of a female-oriented view of the world is the failure of these women to perceive any active working male figure in a TAT story (gamma .52).

Early Sexual-Reproductive Discipline and Instruction

Fewer than half (43.3 percent) the respondents expected menarche when it occurred and more than one-fourth (28 percent) had had no prior information from any source, including friends or reading. Even by the time of the research interview, well past menarche, 28.7 percent had never received any formal instruction about sex or reproduction. More important, 77.3 percent had never had such information offered them by parents or surrogates; only one-fourth had had some discussion about sex and reproduction with mother, and another 11.3 percent with grandparents. For only 8 percent had mother or surrogate been the principal source of information. Among the majority who learned about sex and reproduction from contemporaries, the message was often ambivalent: "They told me I would have to lead that life."

Home discipline in response to the girl's display of sexual interest or concern, reflected in "looking at boys" or asking for information, was recalled as strict and repressive by three-fourths of the respondents, enforced primarily by "flogging" in the experience of almost two-thirds (63.3 percent). As one said, "They were strict-strict . . . never let us go to show or party till we got big . . . Plenty flogging." Another, who lived with a grandmother because her father had deserted her unmarried mother: "If I back to house later than five o'clock she flogged me—to bath, to bed, no food but a glass of milk—she said I was playing with boys." Others explicitly recognized the discrepancy between parental words and deeds: "Father a strict man . . . If I did anything he would beat me . . . When 18 couldn't go anywhere except to church. He say he didn't want me to have a baby too young . . . but him gambling all the time, and he away with women, so when I got pregnant and was afraid, I had nobody to turn to." Or "Our parents led us to believe that men would kill or hurt us or make you pregnant. You had to stay away from them. Mother told me to be careful of men, but didn't explain what she meant. But she had five children with two other men before she came to live with my father and then she had five more."

For half the respondents resentment toward parents, especially mother or (if reared by someone else) surrogate, about lack of sexual-reproductive information was conscious and readily elicited in the interview; for another 14 percent it was easily inferred and was eventually acknowledged with gentle probing.

Almost two-thirds suggested (though rarely explicitly) that they might have been able to learn "what it was like to be a woman" through open communication with their mother rather than through early, unprotected, unpleasurable intercourse and pregnancy. As one woman said, her mother's admonition "Don't have boy friend or you will get pregnant" was understandable but not helpful. Later in the interview she said that if she had been given information when she needed it she would not now, at the age of 22, have three children. Only a few suggested that they successfully resisted parental strictures. For example, "I could thief away now and again and get out." The social transmission of the value of strictness is revealed by the range of women who, despite its obvious failure in their own case, indicated without reflection that they would apply it to their daughters. As one respondent said regarding her 11-year-old daughter's request for sexual information, "I'd flog her . . . She be tryin' turn into a big 'oman." The theme of "trying to become big" is recurrent. In this setting it appears to have two implications. One is that child-rearing patterns are designed to stave off adulthood with its implications of intercourse, pregnancy, and leaving mother for a man. The other fits references to being a "big woman" in terms of ordinary social interactions. This use of the term, though without the specific age and property-owning denotations described in a Maroon community in the St. Mary District (Durant-Gonzalez, 1976), refers to a social status of prestige, power, and respect. In this instance the mother appeared to recognize that her adolescent daughter might be seeking self-esteem and status through her wish for sexual knowledge, intercourse, pregnancy, and a baby of her own. She denies her daughter the sexual knowledge, assuming (despite overwhelming evidence to the contrary) that this denial will preclude attempts to obtain direct experience. The mother's behavior appeared to be designed unconsciously to produce the outcome she was trying consciously to avoid.

Early Experience and the Sexual-Reproductive Career

The 150 respondents may be divided into a majority with little maternal communication (including those reared by grandmothers), an unhappy and conflictful introduction to sexual relations, many sexual partners, and many pregnancies; and a minority with more communication with their mother, a more satisfactory sexual initiation, fewer sexual partners, and fewer pregnancies. Initial coitus for the 17 women never pregnant had occurred on the average two years later (at age 17.4 versus 15.3) than for those ever pregnant, although most had had sufficient unprotected intercourse prior to contracepting to indicate that infertility was a reason for their not having become pregnant. More of these than the 133 ever pregnant (though still only 29.4 percent) had received sexual instruction from their mothers. Only one of the 17 had used a contraceptive device, but four of their partners had used a condom and one had practiced withdrawal at the time of first coitus. The pattern of contraceptive use continued, so that more of the never pregnant than those ever pregnant are current JFPA clients. It is impossible to be certain, however, about the causal significance of various elements in the sequence. Did 5 of the girls choose partners willing to forego "having a baby" by chance, by virtue of their own personalities, or corollary to an open, communicative relationship with their mother? Or did the time afforded by freedom from pregnancy in fact permit the communication with the mother? For the entire group, including the ever pregnant women, it seems apparent that a relationship with a significant maternal figure, sufficiently open to permit some sharing of sexual information, preceded a less strenuous and conflictful sexual-reproductive career than that of the majority of the respondents. These women tended to be older at first coitus; their initial experience was more satisfactory and more likely to involve mutual agreement than force or seduction; and by the time of the interview they had had fewer sexual partners and fewer pregnancies (figure 1).

Although respondents with major information from parents or surrogates had had fewer pregnancies than others of their age group, the largest correlations are with having obtained principal sex knowledge from reading, advertisements, or consultation with professional persons. Use of these impersonal sources (the great majority of respondents could not depend on their mothers) tends to be associated with controlling one's personal fertility, indicated by having had both fewer sexual partners and fewer pregnancies for one's age group. Information seeking seems to represent a coping activity comparable to that involved in managing other aspects of one's life. In contrast, the women who knew least when they first engaged in intercourse became the most sexually and reproductively active. By the time of the interview they were unhappy and angry about their lives. Ninety percent of those who had never used a contraceptive (in contrast with 58 percent of those who had) expressed resentment at their mother's lack of sexual instruction. This awareness of loss of self-determination and of opportunity missed because of early and repeated pregnancy exists despite the rural origins and lack of education of most of the never-contraceptors. Lack of education and especially nonliteracy probably would have made it more difficult for them, in the absence of maternal information, to take advantage of public (usually written) sources of knowledge.

A related set of factors, contributing to age at first coitus and first union, includes three positive matricentric attitudes: belief in the traditional role of the grandmother, in a woman's primary responsibility to mother not mate, and in a predestined "lot" of children (figure 2). These attitudes are less frequent among women who had a communicative relationship with their mothers. Conversely, they are more frequent among women without such communication who were younger at first coitus, first union, and first pregnancy. It is the women who were still matricentrically oriented at the time of the interview who were also angry with their mothers (or surrogates) for withholding the information that would have allowed them to manage the reproductive consequences of their sexuality. The evidence is not of unequivocal rejection of the mother but of ambivalence and conflictful identification conditioned by culture and by idiosyncratic biography.

Male Respondents

In keeping with their better socioeconomic status, most of the males (84.5 percent) were reared in nuclear families by parents

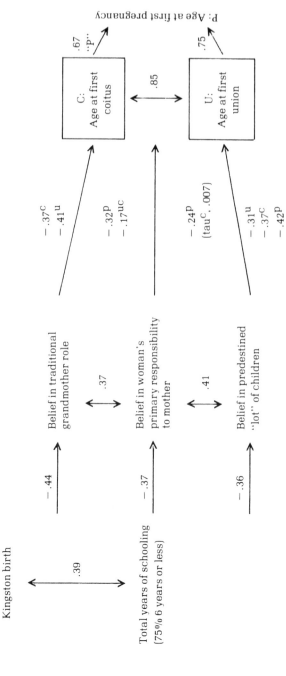

Figure 2. Sociocultural antecedents of age at first coitus, first conjugal union, and first pregnancy of 133 Jamaican women (correlative index, gamma).

or surrogates. Most of the rest (13.4 percent of the total) were reared by mother or grandmother alone. Like the women, very few (9.2 percent) received any positive instruction about sex from mother or father. Unlike them, however, they were not subjected to harshly enforced behavioral restrictions. There was no evidence of the same type of early conflict about sexual behavior or resentment toward parents in this regard. This fits the impression that parents—especially mothers—tend to treat the early sexual explorations of their sons (with their neighbors' daughters) with amused tolerance if not implicit encouragement. This was often hidden, according to the female respondents as well as others in the community, by a thin façade of disapproval. It also seems unlikely that mothers knew about the actual first coital experiences with which their sons began their sexual careers. First coitus was reported at a much earlier age by our male respondents than by the women, with 41.2 percent recalling their initial episodes at between 8 and 10, and 27.5 percent at between 11 and 13 years. Well over two-thirds had apparently had sexual intercourse by the age of 13.

Both sexes appear to have been introduced to sexual intercourse by older and more experienced partners. Although the narrative material from men is scanty, a number of stories are illustrative. For example, one said, "Me teacher said she wanted to see me teapottie [a colloquial word for penis, frequently used with wood and bamboo], so she kept me after school and me show her." Involvement with a teacher was probably rare, but the first partner was almost always someone already known to the boy. Very few, however, had made prior arrangements (over half said it occurred by "chance" or "while playing") and, in contrast to the majority of the women, almost none were already in a courtship or dating relationship with their first partner. Many more men than women could give no particular reason for the event, and few acknowledged the role of curiosity or a need for experience.

Correlations with age at first coitus demonstrate some differences from and similarities with the female respondents. As such, they suggest the possible importance of personal rather than social elements as determinants of some of the observed behavior. Unlike the female sample, no significant correlations emerge within this higher-socioeconomic-status group between age at onset of coital activity and basic indexes of socioeconomic status. Those younger at first coitus, however (or at least reporting earlier sexual experience), tended to have a more traditional attitude toward women. They attributed a submissive attitude to a story heroine in response to a man's request that she have a baby (gamma .29), believed in the traditional role of grandmother (gamma .40), and had a relatively favorable attitude toward mother-headed families (gamma .47). Earlier apparent sexual initiation is, as for the women, related to greater partner diversity according to age (gamma .52), more frequent coitus (gamma .34), and fewer periods of sexual abstinence (gamma .34). Yet unlike the women, there is no relation to number of children, which suggests, as noted earlier, that these sexually active men, even those with traditional male-dominant attitudes who began their coital careers early, are contracepting effectively. They do not attempt to mark each new sexual partnership by the production of a child, and they assume sole responsibility for contraception rather than sharing it with a mate (joint contraceptive decisions vs. younger age at coitus, gamma .28). These findings seem to reflect the special nature of male JFPA clients in terms of the general Jamaican male population.

The Context of Child Rearing and Reproductive Behavior

The context of receiving sexual information and experiencing puberty remains laden with conflict for working-class Jamaican girls. Family life is still dominated in principle, though less in practice, by Victorian ideals of child rearing, part of the missionary legacy. This was noted a generation and a half ago by Kerr (1952) and Clarke (1957) and confirmed by Blake (1961) before contraceptive information and supplies became widely and easily available. It has not changed in consequence of the intense and ubiquitous government contraceptive campaign, in force since 1966 (Brody, 1972, 1974). Attempts to introduce and broaden "family life" teaching in the schools, especially since 1975, have not been in force long enough to permit evaluation of their results. It is probable that the increased outmigration to work in other countries and related changes in values and ideals are affecting sexual-reproductive attitudes, especially those of better educated, urban Jamaicans. The data presented here, however, do not suggest significant differences in daughter-rearing practices in consequence of these attitudes.

The great majority of women respondents, most of them less than 30 years old and living in a context that reinforced the public value of children and motherhood, were reared in circumstances that led them to fear and to distrust the signs of adult femalehood and sexual capacity. Most had "lived" their sexual-reproductive bodies (Merleau-Ponty, 1942) in negative or neutral rather than affirmative terms, despite the fact that preserved virginity was not prominent as a cultural symbol for virtue, goodness, or purity. Their mother had rarely been available for an intimate, supporting, and informing relationship. In these circumstances the private and public, biographical and symbolic meanings of sexuality and reproduction are conflictful. An apparent denial of the body as integral with the experienced self permits its first penetration by another to be attributed to "chance" or to be rationalized as "force." Moreover, the capacity to use one's body as a medium for full self-expression or realization is impaired by a general failure to achieve a harmonious integration of physical with social experience (Douglas, 1970). In these circumstances it is easy for first coitus to symbolize a breaking away from parental restrictions and revenge directed against the mother for prohibiting achievement of a valued status. Without a sense of self as valued and competent, based on an unambivalent maternal identification, capacity to relate mutually with men is impaired. Withdrawal from mutuality is expressed in adherence to matricentric beliefs and a way of engaging with the opposite sex reflected in early and unsatisfactory intercourse, with subsequently high partner diversity and regretted high reproductive performance. This pattern, with its shared symbolic and psychodynamic meanings, has some aspects of a public ritual regularly available for the expression of private needs or the resolution of private conflict.

The likelihood that good communication with one's mother reflects a less ambivalent identification with her is supported by the tendency of women reared by mothers, rather than by other family members or guardians, to be more self-confident in terms of possible careers as well as in dealing with men. They have evidently been more able than most of their peers to utilize their mother as a role model for understanding their own sexuality and reproductive potential and for dealing with men, as well as to gain some sense of themselves as intact, worthwhile persons.

Women responding indifferently to initial intercourse are more apt to subscribe to matricentric beliefs and attitudes and to have little significant communication with their mates. These correlations may represent attitudes and feelings antecedent or consequent to unsatisfactory first coitus. In either event, they suggest not only the perceived centrality of mother as a determinant of seeking and participating in first intercourse, but also the importance of socially transmitted attitudes toward men: their patterns of sexual attitudes and actual relating to men are part of a socially inherited complex of beliefs and values emphasizing the central importance of mothers and the usefulness of men as necessary actors in the creation of babies—or the transformation of girls into mothers.

In Jamaica as elsewhere, first coitus may be considered one of the initial rites of passage marking the transition from childhood to adulthood. It does not, however, appear significant insofar as it involves the loss of virginity, symbolizing sexual purity. It is known to the person him or herself and to the first partner. The first pregnancy is a more significant transitional experience constituting a public announcement to peers, relatives, and others. The often unstable nature of the first sexual-conjugal union makes it unlikely that in Jamaica it symbolizes conjugal and cognatic love in the sense in which Schneider related sexual intercourse in general to American kinship, as a "diffuse, enduring solidarity'' (1973, p. 14). It may signify less a mutual, socially interactive event than an assertion of personal power—the woman's use of the male partner or his use of her to achieve a more valued mature status, to affirm potency, and, in her case in particular, to support a perception of her own body as the key element in child production. Such a perception must be significant for fulfilling the cultural pressure to demonstrate fertility at an early age.

First coitus in Jamaica, and perhaps elsewhere, appears to represent an attempt at conflict resolution, or personal integration. To the extent that the symptomatic character of the act influences its timing, communicative aspects, affective quality, and use or nonuse of contraception, the conflict resolution may be effective. The coital act may permit, without conscious confrontation, the expression of aims or wishes that are marginally acceptable or forbidden in terms of the adolescent girl's intrapsychic conflicts. Its immediate consequences may, however, be immediately adaptive in terms of her current life circumstances even as they ultimately interfere with achieving a stable, reciprocal interrelationship with others. In lower-class Kingston, with its mixture of rural and urban values, the most prominent context-related personal conflicts for postmenarchal girls appear to be those involving the relationship with their mother or surrogate and with men in general. In the maternal relationship these conflicts involve becoming a ''big woman'' in the face of punitive prohibitions and withheld information, and acting out what is forbidden. In relationships with men these conflicts involve a view of men (including contemporary male adolescents) as irresponsible adversaries who may be used for private instrumental purposes but not counted upon as confidants, companions, lovers, or reliable fathers and sources of economic support. In both instances first intercourse (after the crisis of frightening, dangerous menarche has been surmounted) is an act of transition to female adulthood and a way of dealing with the personal conflicts posed by relating to mother or her surrogate and to men. The immediate adaptive value of pregnancy is to gain status in the peer group and some of the previously denied rewards of sexual maturity. The ultimate maladaptive consequences stem from the burden of repeated pregnancies and an increasing number of children with neither a viable emotional or socioeconomic support system.

7 The First Sexual Partnership, the First Pregnancy, and the First Child

Those young girls of Jamaica take warning from me,
Not to chat wit a young mans of a low degree
For he will love you, and he will kiss you
An they will call you their own,
But when de nine months are come, they said 'No me love not I.'

'Oh no, no me love not I,'
But when de nine months are come, they said 'No me love not I.'

Recorded in rural Jamaica and reproduced
with the permission of Olive Lewin

My man no treat me like him use to do,
Like him use to do, like him use to do.
My man no treat me like him use to do,
Because him have a nedda gal wid him.

But if a ketch dat gal a woulda beat her
An disgrace her in every single way.
But if a ketch dat gal a woulda beat her
An disgrace her in every single way.

Recorded in rural Jamaica and reproduced
with the permission of Olive Lewin

Making a Baby

The existence of an open-air market not far from the hospital allowed me to buy fresh vegetables before eight in the morning, when they would be thoroughly picked over. The vendors were friendly and talkative. On an early visit a middle-aged woman, a higgler from the nearby countryside, cautioned me not to drink the water in which I would boil the *ackee-ackee* I was purchasing. "Dem poison," she said. Then she laughed: "You English doctor?" When I told her I was not English but American she replied, "No matter. You docs big brain, but gotta' learn *new* here!" With that she reached beneath the counter and produced an egg. "Dat," she said, "is guinea egg. Eat and you mek baby for sure!"

I thanked her profusely but did not tell her that I had no intention of producing another child. I was not surprised, however, by her message or its personal implications. I was already learning that this is a society in which, despite the high visibility of contraceptives, sexual intercourse still means "making a baby." I was learning, too, that the attribution of fertility is a form of flattery that might be offered a man by a person of either sex. Conversely, deprecatory allusions to poor reproductive capacity are not uncommon, and for men may be linked to implications of femininity and lack of strength and aggressiveness. At its most violent the angry epithet "ras klot" refers to a man as a sanitary pad soiled with menstrual blood. More mildly, the reference may be "Him mama.'"

From the woman's viewpoint the masculine attitude is discussed sarcastically: "Dem tink dat to be man need nothing but drink stout, beat down 'oman, an' leave her wit baby."

I heard the other side of the story from men up and down the socioeconomic scale. In the late afternoon I sometimes went to the shaded outdoor bar of the Senior Commons, half a mile down the campus from the University Hospital. This was a gathering place for graduate students and faculty, predominantly male. As they stood at ease against the counter or lounged at a table with a Red Stripe and a ground-meat "patty," their conversation often turned to women. Its predatory and critical aspects were not unexpected. There was also at times a hint of self-pity, of a sensitivity to lack of appreciation not fundamentally different from that encountered in the United States, but with a slightly sharper edge. Sometimes this would take the form of a wry joke: "What do you think women liked about men before money was invented?" Sometimes it was a direct complaint: "Since my wife's mother moved in with us she doesn't seem to need me any more." The talk would then lead to sexual alternatives. These men as a rule, though, were not interested in producing second or third families. An available woman's interest in having children was exciting but a signal for caution: "Man, she's good, but if you're not careful she's liable to get you so hot that you'll end up giving her a baby!" The youthfulness of potential partners was also viewed as a mixed blessing: "We've just got a new maid in from the country, young and fresh, can't be over 16. I'd like to give it to her and I know she wants it, but you know those country kids. She probably wouldn't want me to use a French letter, and then if she missed her period she'd go to my wife."

Near the market was a tiny bar open to the street. I stopped in often enough to become a familiar face, and the proximity of the University Hospital with its small complement of white physicians from overseas made my presence understandable and acceptable. Among the men here legal marriages were nonexistent. Most conjugal unions appeared to be of a visiting nature except for an occasional older man who was cohabiting. Expressions of sexual desire were similar to those at the Senior Commons, but babies were interpersonal markers and contraception was never spontaneously mentioned. If a particularly nubile young woman walked by, someone might say amidst whistles and sexual comments, "Mon, she ready!" to which another would respond, "Mon, what you know 'bout dat? You not had one baby yet!"

Although there seemed to be an adversary relationship between the sexes, the young girls were not as bitter about men as the older women. I began to realize this during my first two months on the island, when I had a long talk in the privacy of my hospital office with the pregnant 16-year-old sister of a psychiatric patient. She was shy at first, but soon spoke at length about the development of her sister's illness and how anxious it had made her. As we covered the necessary information I learned that my informant was the fourth of nine children living with her mother, both maternal grandparents, and a maternal aunt in a yard in West Kingston, "below the Clock" and "down toward the Spanish Town Road." Her father, she said, had died four years earlier. He had worked hard all his life on a big commercial farm near Spanish Town: "Him nothin' but drudge, cut cane, carry banana." Her grandfather had also worked there but was now an invalid with "bad legs." The adult women did domestic work, "clean up other people's messes," and the children "comin up" had earned whatever money they could. School had not been re-warding and my informant, like her sister, had dropped out of the sixth grade at age 13 shortly after her father's death. Life was not totally unpleasant, though, and she enjoyed helping her mother and looking after the younger children. Her grandmother, who managed the home, was tolerant except for her insistence on going to Sunday school and church. But this changed when, at 14, "out playing I felt me panties wet. Touched me finger, looked down, and saw the blood." Her mother, that night, was dis-tracted after a long day's work and said little. The girl had al-ready known what to expect anyway from her older sisters. Her grandmother, however, changed drastically. "All a sudden she strict-strict, want me in house all the time." The grandmother's lectures about the fact that she could "now have baby" and her stern admonitions to "keep away from boys" were at first fright-ening. The impact soon wore off, however, and was replaced by a slightly guilty pleasure at discussing boys and the nature of having babies with other, now menstruating, girl friends. Her older sisters, one of whom was living with a man for whom she had already had a child, also took her into their confidence. She began to regard her sister's infant with new and increased inter-est. She also began to feel increasingly oppressed, and home, which had once seemed a haven, began to seem a jail to which she returned reluctantly. At the same time she was pleasantly aware that with the development of breasts and hips she was attracting the interested attention of boys. They whistled, stared, and smiled. Then, one day, "there was a boy I knew from school, and we did it." She knew very well that intercourse was the way to "make a baby." Moreover, a friend had told her that "a big vein behind the knee meant I would have children." However, "I never thought about 'the planning' . . . I never expected I would have baby . . . not so quick."

She became pregnant after five months of approximately

weekly intercourse. This was not an occasion for concern. When she "didn't see the period" she was glad "because it would be the first baby and I never sure would have any more." She didn't tell her mother, however, "because she would have quarreled, said I was unruly . . . She found out when she saw me getting fat. She tried to beat me, but she got over it and said, 'Be careful next time. Young girl coming up has better to do than have a baby every year.' " This girl said that she agreed with her mother, but like many others she felt that having the baby was an essential milestone in her life. "You have child and get experience when the baby is born and feel the pain." She also looked ahead to her old age: "Have a baby when you are young so will have when you are old. Granny did and she has us all. Old lady can't get a baby. Wonder what she was doing all the time."

The First Sexual Partnership

Most of the women with whom we talked had "lived" their bodies up to the time of first intercourse as sexually devalued and often hated; they treated their genitals as "bad" or psychologically silent areas. If they recognized the body's pleasure-giving, attractive aspects they were punished by the woman who was their primary gender-role model. An impasse emerged as the maternal figure presented herself, through her own earlier life, as an exemplar of the sexual and reproductive behavior she denied the maturing girl, yet seemed no longer to connect herself with that existence. The impasse could be resolved through sexual action. This meant intercourse, hurriedly at the first opportunity, with little reflection, minimal communication with the partner, and no contraception. It often meant little pleasure or actual physical or emotional discomfort. The sexual act was symbolically important, however: it affirmed the previously denied status of female adulthood. Yet the female initiate tended to exclude from her awareness its reproductive consequences. This exclusion, whether due to ignorance, repression, or deliberate suppression, permits intercourse to be unconsciously used as an attempt to displace the punitive, neglectful mother (or surrogate) as the ruling adult female of the household.

Once the first act of intercourse occurs, a sexual partnership becomes likely. Although the act may be unpleasant and communication minimal or nonexistent, its circumstances and developmental meaning seem to promote rapid bonding. Initial union formation follows initial intercourse as a milestone on the way to motherhood. This means having a partner with whom sexual intercourse and some social exchange can be expected on a regular basis. Ninety-two percent of the first unions in our study group were formed between ages 14 and 20. Approximately 36 percent endured for only one year or less, 20 percent from one to two years, 21 percent for two to four years, and 23.5 percent for more than four years, accounting for many who had had only one union at the time of the research interview. There is a predictably positive correlation between the duration of first union and the respondent's age at the time of the interview, but it is not statistically significant.

Longer first unions are not associated with education, urban birth, or (significantly) with the age when the partnership was formed. This suggests the importance of private, interpersonal factors in compatibility. Positive communication at the time of coitus is positively correlated with the development of an enduring relationship (gamma .28). In addition to initial factors, a commitment to one man promotes more effective communication and reduces the likelihood of other sexual-reproductive relationships and the time available for them. The women whose first sexual partnerships were most enduring were also the most consistent contraceptive users in our population (gamma .47).

As noted earlier, many first unions were terminated without conception. In these or subsequent unions, however, when the first pregnancy did occur the risk of separation from the sexual partner was not reduced. Although women often reported that their man had asked them to "have a baby for him," this request did not usually motivate her to have unprotected intercourse. It did become important, however, once she found herself pregnant, especially for the first time. At that point she often felt that she was indeed "making a baby for" her partner. If he deserted her, her feelings of loss and anger were doubly intense.

More than 40 percent of the couples separated before their

first child was one year old. Over half of these separations occurred before delivery, generally at about the sixth month, when
the pregnancy became visible and the girl began to be less interested in regular intercourse. Separation is difficult for the pregnant girl who has left her mother's home when it involves a re-
criminatory "I told you so" from family members to whom she
must now return. It is especially upsetting when she had after all
been deserted by the man "for" whom she had had the baby in
the first place. Feelings were equally intense if she had left him
because of discovery of his simultaneous involvement with other
women who had also sometimes had children for him. On the
other hand, separation in some instances was initiated by the girl
—usually abetted by her mother—who felt that she was too
young to assume the conjugal relationship or that she did not
wish to interrupt her schooling.

The man's conflicting feelings are revealed both by desertion
(in seven instances through emigration) and by denial of paternity (in six cases). The earlier wish for a child, however, seemed
not to disappear; either he or his family contributed to the child's
support once the flurry of denial had passed.

The failure of the first child to keep the couple together or to
bond the man to the woman who had had it "for" him is indicated
by the finding that approximately two-thirds of the conjugal pairs
were separated by the time the child was five. This proportion is
probably higher in the population at large, for only half of the intact first couples in the sample had children who were older. The
child seems relatively unimportant as a symbol and manifest of
the relationship, despite the expressed request and intent to have
a baby "for" the man. On the contrary, coitus and parenthood
seem, in retrospect, more important for the man and woman as
individuals rather than as members of a partnership.

The First Pregnancy

Approximately one-fifth of the respondents conceived within
their first menstrual cycle after beginning regular intercourse;
that is, after forming an initial sexual partnership. The majority,

sometimes by then with a second partner, were pregnant within six months. The median age of first pregnancy was 16, and it had occurred for almost all by their twenty-first birthday. Successive pregnancies followed quickly: the second and third for most by age 25 (with a median age for the second of 21), and the fourth, fifth, or sixth by 29.

Their early age at first pregnancy was for some a matter of conscious regret. For others it was the expression of an urgent wish. Many greeted it with pride and pleasure as a visible mark of status. Most, though, offered an opportunity, expressed mixed feelings, which can often be related to their feeling about first intercourse and becoming a "big woman." These mixed feelings also resulted from earlier, repeated observations of the pregnancies of women around them: adult women, often unhappy with yet another pregnancy, were at least left alone by their relatives. Age-mates, flogged and vilified by mothers or older maternal caretakers, were admired and envied by peers. In time, however, they, too, became large, stretched, and uncomfortable. And by that time they, too, had been accepted and, without the anger of their mothers to deal with, were left to confront their own feelings. All were apprehensive about the pain of delivery. Most also understood that many friends whose male partners had urged them to become pregnant had been left alone. First the man's attentions had declined: with late pregnancy "him couldn't fool with them no more." Then, after expressing joy at having become a father, especially if "it first baby for him," he visited less and less frequently and finally disappeared. His source of satisfaction was "having" the baby, not rearing it.

The stories behind the data summaries are varied, but most confirm the common points: ambivalence toward mother, ambivalence toward the male partner, early denial of the reproductive consequences of intercourse, and a fundamental wish to become a mother despite awareness of the real life problems that it entails.

One woman remembered that she went to a clinic at age 18 having missed two periods after six months of unprotected intercourse. She was shocked and frightened, thinking that she was "too young" and wondering how her mother would react, when the doctor said, "You are making a baby." Then she realized she had known all along that she could become pregnant and simply had not bothered to obtain a contraceptive: "I felt I was taking a chance . . . I wanted the experience for myself." When she found that she was indeed "making a baby . . . that's when I began to experience life for myself . . . It pain . . . You don't always get what you want, and the baby-father can go away . . . but you have the baby and you know what it is like." After a second baby, she and her boy friend discussed marriage, but her mother said she would never consent because she didn't like the man. She has since had two more children by a second man and hopes for eventual marriage.

Some women recall becoming adult rather than just obtaining "experience" as part of the meaning of first pregnancy. One, for example, missed her period at 16 after several months of irregular coitus. Although she had used no contraception "because I didn't know about it," she was sufficiently aware of the connection between coitus and pregnancy to fear telling her mother about it. Then her mother noticed that she was not eating and took her to a doctor, who confirmed the pregnancy. The mother flogged her repeatedly, stating over and over that she "did not want any more big women"—meaning adult, reproductively capable, females—"in the house." A spontaneous abortion occurred within the month. The respondent was relieved but at the same time resentful of her mother, who "wanted to keep me small." Despite her conscious statement that she did not want to become pregnant again, she had four babies by two other men in the next few years. She still lives at home with her mother and maintains a visiting union with her current mate, whom her mother considers "too wild" to be a reliable cohabiting partner.

Antecedents and Consequences of First Pregnancy

The practical significance of the first sexual partnership—usually a visiting arrangement—is to facilitate and regularize sexual intercourse. The ages of these two closely related events—first intercourse and first union—account for approximately half of the variation among respondents in age at first pregnancy (figure 3). The rest can be attributed to differences in the frequency and timing of intercourse, organic deviation or illness in the two partners, and, least of all, contraceptive use.

Both contraceptive use and age at first intercourse and union reflect the nature of the woman's earlier relationships. An affectively positive maternal identification seems especially important. The early receipt of sexual information from mother or surrogate was reported by only a minority of the women and tended to be followed by meaningful communication with the first partner in intercourse. Girls with the options and security provided by sexual knowledge, supported by their mothers in their developing status as adult females, are able to begin their sexual-reproductive careers in more positive and less traumatic fashion than others. They select more open men as partners, and insist on some mutual sharing of feelings and ideas as well as bodies. Perhaps in consequence their first unions are more enduring (figure 4), and they more frequently use contraceptives; both factors contribute to a delayed first pregnancy. This first union may help set a pattern for later ones. Women older at first pregnancy by an initial partner more often discussed contraceptive use with him (figure 4) and with their current mate as well (figure 5). More dramatically, being younger at first pregnancy results in a predictable sexual-reproductive career. Women who conceived earlier in adolescence went on to become involved with more visiting male partners than those who first conceived later. By the time of the research interview they not only had had more pregnancies but also had been impregnated by more men than other women with the same number of pregnancies (figure 3). The younger the woman at the time of first pregnancy, the more likely she was to have had a second pregnancy by a second man and a third pregnancy by a third man, with none of whom she had discussed contraception (figure 5).

There are, however, many exceptions to this pattern. Contraceptive use and the acquisition of new male partners may be initiated, continued, or stopped at any point in a woman's reproduc-

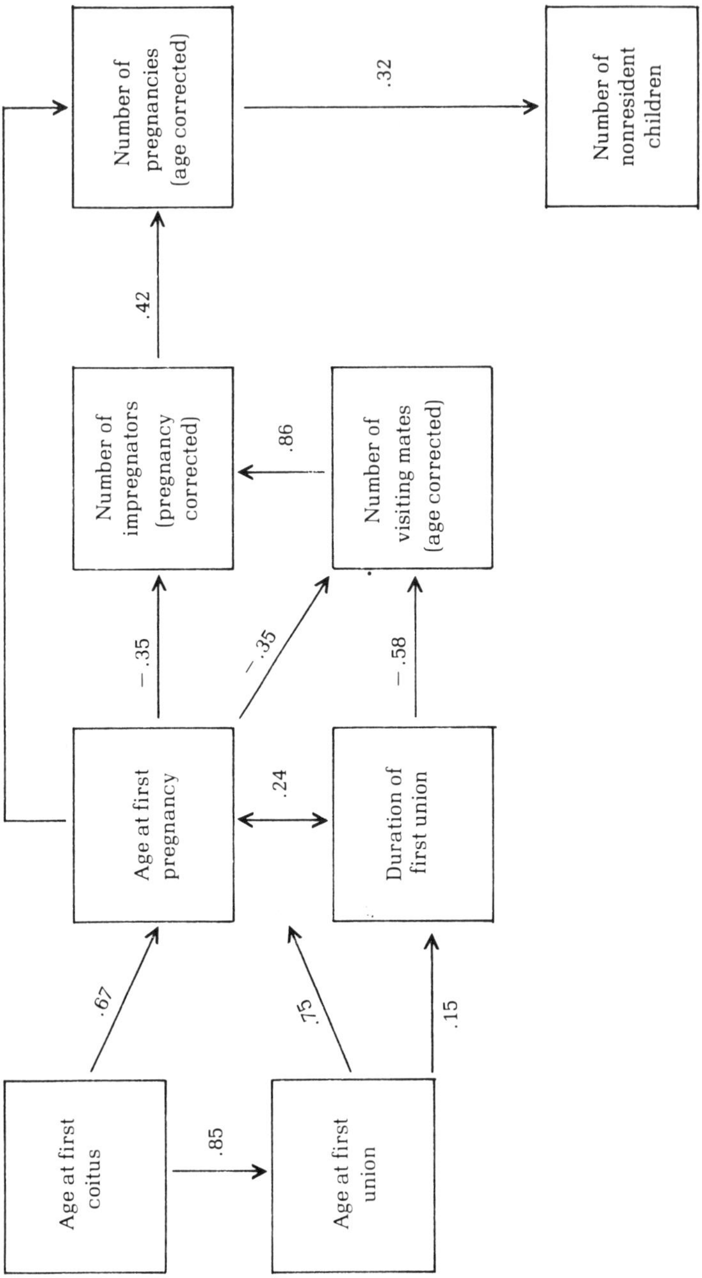

Figure 3. Path from age at first coitus/pregnancy to partner diversity and reproductive performance of 133 Jamaican women (correlative index, gamma).

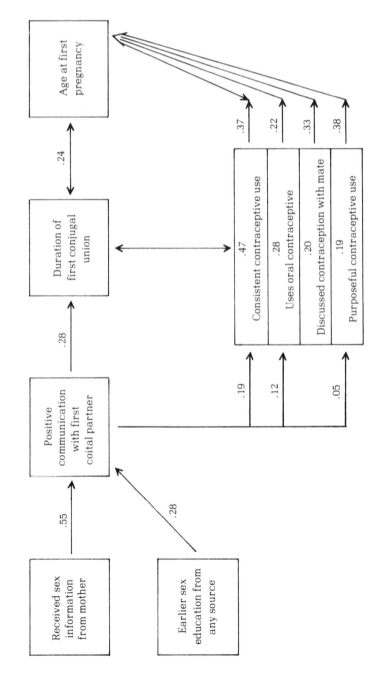

Figure 4. Early information and communication in relation to duration of first conjugal union and age at first pregnancy of 133 Jamaican women (correlative index, gamma).

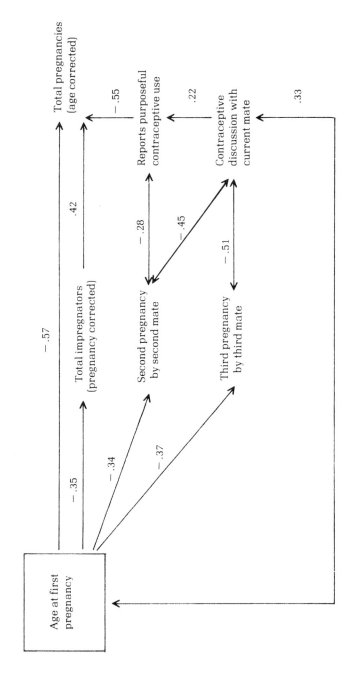

Figure 5. Postcedents of age at first pregnancy of 133 Jamaican women (correlative index. gamma). Age at interview: range 16–47. mean 26.5. 80% age 30 or less.

tive career regardless of her having started to reproduce late under favorable circumstances. This career involves repeated sexual intercourse and conjugal unions as well as pregnancies and deliveries.

An example of individual variation is provided by a woman who had been given sexual-reproductive information by the aunt and uncle with whom she lived. Her first experience of intercourse at age 18 was accompanied by good communication with her partner. They formed a visiting union, and her boy friend, who had had some college agreed to her request that he use condoms. After three years, however, he went abroad to study and, despite his promises of marriage, finally stopped corresponding. She was very lonely and began another alliance. Although her new boy friend was a teacher, he refused to use condoms and gave no reason. She didn't know what to do and "didn't want to drive him off," so she continued intercourse. Within a year she was pregnant, beginning a career eventuating in several children by two men.

An example of muted conflict and communication failure even after considerable experience and with an educated partner is seen in the interaction between a respondent who was already a mother and her second mate. She was 22 at the time; he was a 35-year-old unmarried school teacher who had one child of his own. Contraception was his idea and he used both a condom and foam tablets. After about five months, however, she noticed that sometimes he forgot his condoms: "I knew I could get pregnant and I didn't especially want another baby . . . It was a chance"; but it never occurred to her to refuse coitus, to obtain her own contraceptives, or to question him. Despite repeated sexual intercourse her solitude remained unbroken: "I didn't tell him my life story. Didn't think it was a good thing to talk about with him."

More typical is a story of having been to a school party at age 15 and accompanying a 17-year-old friend to his home to discover that his mother was out: "I didn't want to do it, but he wanted to. I didn't want to have a baby but he said he would take care of everything. I didn't know what he would do, but was afraid to ask, so I didn't say more. Anyway, I knew I was taking a chance

. . . but I just wondered what it was like . . . thought it would have to happen sometime." Coitus did not become pleasurable although they "had it" five or six times in the ensuing 18 months. They hardly spoke with each other and she never brought up the contraceptive issue again, but she concluded that he was in fact doing nothing. By then, however, her older sister and friends had babies and "I thought it would be nice if I had one . . . Mother would be angry, but I knew she would take it and care for it."

The women fell naturally into two groups, differentiated initially by useful communication with their mother about sex. The minority who had such communication tended to be older at first coitus and to have positive communication with the first sexual partner and a longer first union. They engaged in more contraceptive discussion with their mates, used contraceptives more purposefully, and in consequence were older when they first became pregnant. The majority had little or no useful communication with their mothers about sex or reproduction. They had early intercourse with little discussion with their partners, did not contracept, and became pregnant early.

Failure to Contracept

Reproductive Knowledge

The lack of knowledge in this urban population after several years of exposure to an intense informational campaign is impressive. Despite the selection of two-thirds on the basis of their being family planning clients, less than half the women had any basic understanding of the reproductive process, and only one-fourth had a conventional knowledge of contraception or abortion. Approximately one-third said they had learned what they did know from a friend, approximately one-fourth from nurses or other professionals (as in the JFPA), and only a few from the media campaigns.

Although there is no significant correlation between possessing reproductive knowledge and contraceptive use or fertility, the ignorance implied by its lack is a significant aspect of the contexts of first and later pregnancies and their possible meaning.

Psychological resistance—excluding available information through denial—is suggested by the fact that only 10 percent of the respondents (two-thirds of whom are JFPA clients) described themselves as unambivalently in favor of contraception.

Most of the 120 women who had ever used a technical contraceptive method first did so between the ages of 17 and 23, and almost all had tried it by age 30. Almost none had employed a method prior to their first pregnancy (table 11). Only one-fifth of the group of 150 attributed failure to contracept to their own or their mate's conscious and explicit wish to have a baby. For the rest the reasons given for not contracepting are vague, summarized as inertia, nonspecific apprehension, and taking the path of least resistance. Some specific complaints, especially of pain or discomfort, were noted by almost one-fourth upon detailed questioning. Bleeding, inconvenience, unreliability, the risk of sexual dysfunction, and similar objections were each noted by a few women, many of whom had also complained of pain, sometimes in the abdomen or pelvis but also elsewhere in the body. For five of the women belief in a foreordained "lot" was involved in early unprotected intercourse: "If you are going to have a certain amount of children, you might as well start 16 or 17, then out and done."

As women became successively pregnant they tended more often to employ contraceptives. The consistent, though small, increase in contraception with successive pregnancies suggests an increasing wish to avoid having still another baby. Yet almost three-fourths of the women with four or more pregnancies had made no prior effort to interfere with the reproductive consequence of intercourse. Even more impressive is the fact that lack of knowledge and fear continue relatively unabated over successive pregnancies as reasons for not contracepting.

Many individual responses suggested the existence of a substratum of knowledge, ignored by the respondent on the basis of ideas that she actually recognized as unreliable. As one woman put it, she knew she was "taking a chance" by having intercourse without contraception, but "because we never did it more than once a week I didn't think I would have a baby." Others said they

Table 11. Reasons for nonuse or ineffective contraception prior to successive pregnancies of 133 Jamaican women.

Pregnancy number	Number of women pregnant	Not contracepting	No reason Difficult Inconvenient Involved risk	Lack of general knowledge associated with fear of consequences[a]	Wanted pregnancy or opposed to contraception (subject or mate)
1	133	94.0%	44.5%	34.3%	21.0%
2	102	83.4	38.6	42.5	18.8
3	78	81.9	40.2	40.2	19.4
4	61	78.7	40.0	43.3	16.6
5	40	72.5	41.0	43.5	15.3
6	22	68.7	45.4	45.4	9.0

a. All but 6 were knowledgeable about types and availability of technical methods.

didn't expect to become pregnant because they were "too small" or "not a big woman yet" or more often that they simply "didn't think about anything like that." Some reported their boy friends' objections; one had said that a condom "gives cancer. I didn't really believe it, but decided that if a baby would come, there was nothing I could do about it."

Others who said that they "didn't know about such things" or "I didn't hear about that as yet" seemed to have been exposed to information without receiving it. As one woman reported, neither she nor her first mate had wanted a baby, but they did nothing to prevent it. She listened to the radio all the time, but could not recall having heard advertisements for family planning. Although she lived within walking distance of the East Street clinic she did not become aware of its existence until she had three babies to care for. "Somehow we just never talked about it." When she did become pregnant for the first time, the thought of abortion "passed through my mind, but that not right . . . 'The control' is okay because you can remove it if you want another."

A more striking example is a woman reared by a religious aunt after her mother's early death. She attended a Catholic school and remembers clearly that when she was 13, at about the time of her menarche, one of the nuns instructed the class about reproductive physiology. She knew that sexual intercourse could lead to pregnancy and was aware of the family planning posters. Yet when, at age 17, her boy friend (who stayed overnight at her house because of a heavy rainstorm) initiated sexual intercourse, "the thought of becoming pregnant didn't even cross my mind." They continued to have coitus approximately once weekly for about six months before she conceived. She was frightened and upset because it would interfere with her educational plans, but he was happy and wanted to get married. Finally she told her aunt, who agreed with her that she would be better off and have more freedom later if she did not become tied to a man. She refused further intercourse with her boy friend and was very relieved when, about two months later, she had a spontaneous abortion. The boy friend, in contrast, had been looking forward to fatherhood and was disappointed. With the detachment offered by the terminated pregnancy, she wondered why she had allowed herself to risk pregnancy, concluding that she had been blindly dependent on him—he was five years older and experienced. When she asked him why he "had not used protection," he replied that "it would throw him off" and also that it "would not be fair" to him if she used something. She obtained a pamphlet on contraception from the clinic and showed it to him, but he responded, "These things are for people who have six children, not for someone who doesn't have any." Since it became clear that he would not cooperate and she wanted to resume their sexual relationship, without telling him she began using an oral contraceptive six months before the research interview. "Someday," she said, she "will get around to talk to him about it, but not just now."

The Value of Children, Especially Daughters

A socially inherited wish to prove one's fertility is suggested by the respondents' unequivocally positive feelings about child production. Most are, without apparent conflict, negative about being unable to have a baby. They are similarly positive about having a child to care for. The pattern is revealed in one country-born woman's comment: "Family planning keeps woman from having children when don't want them. But I always wondered if I was going to have any. Was afraid that would get old and not. Began thinking, 16 or 17, didn't want to get to 18 or 19 without them, especially after I saw them having children at 13 or 14." As another said, "If you are a barren woman all your days wasted." The wish for a daughter figured in the retrospective accounts of approximately half the women and was invariably related to expectations of companionship in old age. The economic element was often implied but rarely explicit. Fear of personal isolation seemed more acute. For example: "Children should just love their mother and grandmother when they get older; your daughter comb your hair. I will look after my mother, which of my children will do for me?" Or "If you are old and no one to care for you, you expect to live with your daughter. They would see I am looked after properly. It is better having girls, you can stay with them and play with your grandchildren."

One woman stated directly, "I don't like boys. When you get old you have a daughter come around . . . like how nice my mother feel when she sees us . . . A daughter go talk with you, help you, especially when you are sick. When a son big he just big and leave his mother and find a woman for himself."

Sometimes the gender reference is less explicit: "Children are a great comfort to you and help when you become old. When there was nobody when my mother took sick, my brother sent me a telegram to come. He had to work, but I stayed with her for two months. You should not have two children unless you can afford it. But if you can have one and don't, it really not right. Some old people say they wish they would die because they have nobody." This theme was widespread. For example: "I would not feel happy to know that I could not have a child. I would just feel that after my mother and father dead I would be in the world alone . . . not no one." Another, anticipating the future: "I feel years when older, you have a child, you can call out, please make me cup of hot water, come comb my hair for me . . . and she come."

The theme of sickness is also frequent. For example: "Not like it didn't have even one child. If I am sick and all those things, want somebody for myself to help me clean my house, spread my bed, go for water." Only rarely was money a specific focus of attention: "Maybe you will be sick and can't move. Child will get me some money or something like that. Maybe you can't pay the rent or something like that." Several said that if they were sterile they would adopt a baby. As one said, "To have somebody around keeps people together . . . It's good to have a child, a daughter, you can take care of her and she of you. You don't need to reproduce her yourself. She still you child."

Distrust of sons, not often explicated, seems linked to distrust of men in general. For example: "Here young boys don't think, they just run up and down. Maybe it's in their nature." Or "Them not want to settle down or care anyone. Say only foolish people and who have money get married. Can't count on them when old." Or "Jamaican men not think about life. Just see a girl you know, and she looks nice and they gone."

Occasionally women will become pregnant a second or third time hoping for a daughter. One woman, for example, had wanted a girl: "I really didn't want a second baby, and mother would never consent to my marrying the baby-father because she didn't like him, but I went ahead and did." When the second child turned out to be a boy she broke up with her partner. Within three months she gave the baby to an unmarried paternal aunt who wanted a child to rear, moved out of the parental home into a room of her own, and established a new visiting union with a man who lived nearby. Because she did not want a third baby she obtained a diaphragm from the East Street clinic. Her new partner, however, objected, saying that he "felt something funny" during intercourse. He said, "It better for you to have the baby . . . Family plannings do more harm than help to you . . . It will hurt your health." Because she "felt close to him" and "it was his first child" she allowed herself to become pregnant. She had expected him to be elated, so she was tremendously let down when all he said upon learning that she "didn't see her period" was "okay." This disappointment contributed to her decision after the child was born to start taking the pill. She took it irregularly, however, because she thought it made her feel nauseated. When, to her dismay but not intense surprise, she became pregnant for a fourth time she consulted a physician about an abortion: "It was getting so my experience of life was not pleasant." The doctor wanted $30. She thought the price "too dear . . . I could have used it to prepare things for the baby." Later she abandoned the whole idea because "I don't care what happen in life, I not going to throw the baby away. I going to bring it . . . and that was a girl so I was happy with it."

The Quality of the First Pregnancy

Personal Feelings

The first pregnancy was uncomfortable and a source of ambivalence for almost two-thirds of the respondents. Another 10 percent reported themselves as indifferent or neutral. Life was difficult when parents quarreled and perhaps threatened expulsion from the home. The man "for" whom the girl had the baby often left her. With successive pregnancies the relationship with the "baby-father" usually became more stable. The proportion of negative feelings during the nine months diminished only slightly, however, and was replaced by indifferent rather than positive responses.

One representative experience began when the respondent was 18. Her mother had gone to the country, leaving her with her younger siblings. A boy four or five years her senior whom she had known "for a long time, found me there . . . I was afraid and didn't want to do it, but he held me." She was afraid to tell her mother for fear of being flogged, but confided in her sister, who did report it. The mother talked to the boy, "who said if I had a baby, he would stand by me . . . He said he wanted to marry me, but I didn't want to leave my mother and experience life."

The next time they had intercourse she enjoyed it and the boy began to visit her weekly. Although she did not want a baby, she "decided to take a chance" and they used no contraception. Her partner was happy because she did not insist on it: "He want a child so he can say he is a big man." Within six weeks she "didn't see" her period. Despite her earlier willingness to "take a chance" she felt very sad, more so after the doctor confirmed the pregnancy. She wanted to please her partner and he treated her well and started giving her money as soon as she was pregnant. Nonetheless she often felt angry and "quarreled him." She cried frequently and had a "bad feeling and threw up" during the first six months. Toward the end, however, she began to feel calm and look forward to the baby's arrival.

In some seemingly conflict-laden cases, on the other hand, pregnancy was uneventful. A girl was "forced" at age 17 by a boy she had known for a year. She told no one because her parents "would quarrel and flog me . . . Father flogs for every little thing." After missing her next period, she had her pregnancy confirmed at Jubilee Hospital. She was not acutely distressed, however, and immediately obtained a tonic "for the baby," which she took for two months before telling her mother. Her mother was upset but helpful and arranged for her to live with a cousin; when she moved out, however, her father had to know why. He was enraged to learn she was pregnant and told her never to come back. At that point the "boy friend" who had "forced" her decided he wanted to marry her. He went to see her mother about it, but neither she nor her daughter was interested: "Mother didn't think much of him and anyway I wanted to finish school." After an uneventful pregnancy and delivery, this woman's father, like most others, "forgave" her. She moved back into her parents' house with her child and resumed her schooling. Neither parent liked her partner, and "I didn't care that much so I told him not to come back." She remained in her parents' home but for the past five years had had a visiting union with another "boy friend," for whom she had had one child. The child lived with the boy friend's mother. After her second child she obtained an IUD. Her boy friend said that it interfered with his pleasure, but she thought this was not true and that he really objected because he wanted more children.

Attitudes toward Successive Pregnancies

The special significance of the first pregnancy and first child was confirmed by marked changes in the respondents' attitudes with the accumulation of pregnancies and children. The more pregnancies a woman had in comparison with others of the same age, the less likely she was to feel positively about motherhood (gamma $-.46$), child care (gamma $-.30$), or pregnancy (gamma $-.43$). She was also less likely to be unequivocally negative about being sterile (gamma $-.42$): the idea of being "barren" no longer evoked feelings of despair, loneliness, or shame. In contrast, all but one of the 17 never-pregnant women affirmed the value of motherhood and were negative about sterility.

Individual accounts of second and ensuing pregnancies varied considerably. Most referred to the male partner's wishes for a large family and some to their own parents' desires for grandchildren. Others expressed obvious ambivalence. For example: "If I had no children it might be better . . . a lot of heartaches. But having children is something real nice." Or "I get pleasure from the baby, but if I only had two, they might get a little more food to eat and you can save more money to school them."

For many, the diminishing pleasure in births after the first is related to progressive disillusionment with men: "Jamaican man just want to give woman a lot of babies and just run off and leave them." Or "He might have been glad because it [her third] was his first child, but don't count on anything anymore."

Fertility-Related Attitudes

Attitudes toward being pregnant, motherhood, giving birth, child care, and being fertile reflected life experience up to the time of the interview. The views that perpetuate the inclination to have large families were modified with stressful reproductive and parental experience. By the time such experience accumulated, however, the new reproductive career was well under way and a new family had already been formed.

Women who by the time of the research interview were still positive about being pregnant were those with a relatively favorable context of development. They had learned about sex from parental figures, especially their mother, around the time of menarche. Subsequently they were able to talk in a personally meaningful way with their first partner in intercourse. These women discussed contraception with their current mate, had a more consistent and satisfying conjugal union, and tended to be more socioeconomically advantaged within the group. In contrast, those who felt negative tended already to have had many sexual partners, pregnancies, and children, some of whom they had had to "pass on" to others to rear.

Feelings about infertility are intense among younger, particularly rural, women and are part of their folklore. The respondents seemed ambivalent about it, especially those with many pregnancies, children, and sexual partners. Of the 150 women, however, 125 expressed themselves negatively about being infertile, sterile, or barren. Of these, 103 said it would make them feel unfulfilled or inadequate.

Valuing the ability to have children or feeling unfulfilled about the inability to do so, like remaining positive about pregnancy, is correlated with favorable developmental and current experiences and indications of personal competence. Literacy (gamma .40), ability to draw a human figure (gamma .34), and having higher occupational aspirations (gamma .45) are associated with valuing fertility but not pregnancy. These seemed to be associated in the more integrated women with the best life experience who had the least actual need for children as companions or sources of economic security.

Conversely, less favorable early and current experiences are associated with not valuing the ability to have children so highly, or not perceiving sterility or childlessness in such unpleasant or devalued ways. These include the circumstances associated with having grandmother in the home and having had children with inconsistent male support. The women with the least favorable early sexual experience seemed to value children more as a means to emotional or economic security rather than as ends in themselves. Whether this was true at the time of first pregnancy seems doubtful. Some women, able to relate warmly to the interviewer despite a stressful past life, were still able to view reproduction in terms of choice. As an unmarried 24-year-old mother of three remarked, "If you can support and school your children, that nice. If you can't, it not nice and you should wait till you can." Reared by grandmothers and believing in their traditional role, they probably considered an early demonstration of fertility important. But it is precisely these women who were more vulnerable to experiences that tend to have the opposite effect, to disillusion them about the value of fertility. Such experience, leading to early and frequent pregnancy under undesirable circumstances and therefore to being less negative about infertility, was more prevalent among the less advantaged respondents, who tended to retain their traditional beliefs.

Thus, fertility-related attitudes simultaneously reflect a basic, developmentally nurtured view of life on one hand and the often burdensome consequences of adult reproductive experience on the other. These last are suggested by the sexual-reproductive decisions attributed by respondents to story heroines. Responses

to specific stories are not significantly correlated with socioeconomic or cultural status; but more of the never-pregnant women
said a story heroine would abort an unwanted pregnancy. Fewer,
however, said they would do so themselves. On one hand, 15
JFPA clients among the 17 respondents who had never conceived
seemed more autonomous, as is suggested by their later first
coitus and use of contraception. On the other, 14 of these JFPA
clients had had and the two Manley never-pregnant patients
were continuing to have unprotected intercourse. They may well
have felt their failure to conceive as a personal failure. Although
most were then—after unproductive sexual intercourse—using
contraceptives, it is not unlikely that they would not do so consistently or for a prolonged period. Similarly, a slightly higher proportion of those never pregnant said that a never-pregnant girl
would reject a man's proposal that she have a child for him.
Fewer, however, had a heroine with children reject child support
in return for having another "for" a man. Almost one-third, a
considerably higher proportion than among the ever pregnant,
were unsure what the heroine should do in the latter situation. In
contrast to those with children, they seemed to be weighing the
realistic advantages of accepting support in return for producing
another baby. They were less skeptical than the others of the
man's good intentions, more optimistic about his being a help
rather than a burden, and less concerned about the added responsibilities of another child. The degree to which this uncertainty may have reflected an ambivalent wish to have a baby is a
matter of conjecture.

The general dislike for abortion, coupled with a fundamentally
positive feeling for having babies, is reflected in some story responses. A heroine impregnated for the first time by a man who
says he will not support her or the baby would, according to more
than three-fourths of the respondents, go ahead nonetheless and
"have the baby for him." Almost two-thirds of the respondents
would themselves have done the same. But only 40 percent perceived a heroine who already has a child as ready to go ahead
and have yet another baby "for" a new man in return for his
promised support for those she already has; and even fewer of

the respondents would themselves have done the same. Many would have liked first a period of support as a token of good intentions, and several others would have accepted the man's support while secretly using a contraceptive. Almost everyone drew the line against a pregnancy for a man in favor of staying in school—a value that in real life is honored mainly in the breach.

The First Child

Although the first pregnancy is acknowledged reluctantly, often with protestations of surprise, initially turbulent feelings tend to be replaced in time with a sense of anticipated achievement. The adolescent begins to think of herself less as a girl who has missed her period and more as someone on the threshold of new status, a future mother. The first child was received with unequivocal pleasure by almost three-quarters of the respondents. As one said, "I was proud to see my baby." The theme of pride in personal ability is prominent: "I was proud to be a mother." Or "It felt good to know I was able." Or "It made me feel proud." In no instance was there any mention of the father's role or a designation of the new baby as "ours."

The next child and those that came after it, however, are received differently. The now experienced mothers are less happy and self-satisfied with succeeding babies. Positive responses dropped sharply with the second delivery; negative and indifferent responses rose. Major sources of dissatisfaction were unhappiness with the "baby-father," economic insecurity, and, with accumulating children, developing restrictions upon personal freedom and opportunity. Explicitly negative reactions remained relatively low—it seemed less acceptable to say that one did not in fact want or appreciate the baby one had conceived and carried about inside one—but by the third delivery, indifferent responses to the new baby had almost tripled. Indifference, a form of withdrawal, is a more prevalent subjective expression of disaffection than is direct engagement with anger, disgust, or an explicit wish to reject a potential relationship that is both a direct and a symbolic constraint on personal freedom. Later negative reactions also included some disturbances associated with still-births, which rose with successive pregnancies, and disappointments in the baby's gender.

Passing On

One form of rejection that, because it is institutionalized, need not involve confrontation with a wish to reject one's baby is "passing on." The practice of passing on a child to a relative or some other person to rear is widespread in Jamaica. Clarke (1957) found that an average of 18 percent of the children in three communities lived with foster parents. Almost half of those from the poorest community lived with nonkin, but all from the most prosperous were with relatives. An underrepresentation of children less than 14 years old in 425 lower-income Kingston households (R. G. Smith, 1962) was attributed to the fact that many women leave children with country relatives when they come to the city to find work; others, already dwelling in the city, send children "back" to these relatives when they feel pressed for their care by lack of time and resources. More recently, "passing on" has been described as a means of dealing with problem children. "Leaving a child in a borrowed toilet, at a busy street corner, in someone's car . . . are only more extreme forms of passing on to a father, a cousin, or a woman who needs a child to help her in the market. This is essentially what happens with the child in the grand-mother and extended families . . . [where] parents have passed on certain aspects of their caring to a member of their kin group" (Brodber, 1974, p. 49).

Of 131 mothers with living children, 57 percent had passed on a total of 121, usually in infancy, to others to rear. Almost one-third had given up their entire family to date, and 60 percent had passed on half or more of their children. Of these children almost half were first-born. The prevalence of passing the first-born on to others reflects the relative instability of initial unions and the youth of first-time mothers. The significance of the act as a cultural pattern for deprived women is suggested by the fact that almost one-third of the second and third and one-fifth of the fourth children were also given to others to rear.

In the majority of cases the young mother gave her baby to a female member of her own family. In a few instances the father's mother, occasionally in anticipation of a rupture of the union, explicitly requested the child. Together almost 58 percent of the passed-on children were reared by grandmothers.

In the great majority of instances the new home was located away from Kingston in a rural area, and after the child was transferred the tie with the biological mother became weak. As one woman said, "My mother took Junior when he was a baby because I had no man to turn to and had to work to take care of myself. Now he looks to her like his mummy." Almost three-fourths of the women visited their passed-on children less than once monthly; six children were never visited, and 25 only once a year or even less often. Except in two cases, these 31 never or rarely visited children were with their fathers or paternal relatives.

Women with passed-on children can be viewed as a group with some common characteristics (table 12). These include a tendency to have had several sexual partners, more children than average for their age, and a currently noncohabiting union. These features fit their less advantaged socioeconomic and familial backgrounds, reflected in more traditional and matricentric attitudes. These attitudes and relatively strong ties with "the country" may contribute to a readiness to utilize other female relatives to rear their children. But they may also be part of a cluster associated with less interpersonal, and possibly less child-rearing, competence. Thus, they tended to draw immature, poorly formed, and distorted human figures. Possible openness to any source of help, either in consequence of the crisis or the factors contributing to crisis, is suggested by their tendency to have a story heroine assent to a white man's proposal to keep her in return for sexual relations.

These characteristics tend to support the impression that passing on in Jamaica can be understood largely in terms of "crisis fostering" and, furthermore, that a rural background associated

Table 12. Gamma correlations between characteristics of 131 Jamaican mothers and their having passed children on; 61 women (46.9 percent) had passed on no children, 38 (29.2 percent) had passed on one child, and 32 (24.4 percent) had passed on more than one.

Characteristics	Correlation
Conjugal-reproductive history	
Number of impregnators (per pregnancy with two or more children)[a]	.48
Number of visiting mates (per 10 sexually active years)	.41
Number of pregnancies (below, median, or above, by age)	.32
Contracepted to delay initial or to space later births	−.28
Stability of current conjugal union (married, cohabits, visits, broken)	−.27
Socioeconomic status	
Piped water in dwelling	−.38
Years of schooling	−.30
Cultural beliefs	
Belief in traditional role of grandmother	.46
Belief in "lot" of children	.35
Personal competence-autonomy	
Draw-a-person score	−.44
Details on draw-a-person	−.31
Story heroine rejects white man's proposal to keep her	−.30
Able to acquire sex knowledge from reading or professionals (teachers, nurses)	−.26
Acknowledges affective element in TAT story	−.24
Early history	
Urban (vs. small town vs. rural) birth	−.32
Grandmother in home more than half the time before age 15	.35

a. 101 had two or more children.

with traditional attitudes may make this a more acceptable way of coping. The degree to which solutions of this sort to repeated and expectable stressful situations can be institutionalized is seen in the matter-of-fact comments of many respondents. As one unemployed woman whose mate had just left her said on discovering her second pregnancy, "Me mother can take the baby . . .

She still hale and hearty!'' This respondent's first child, whom she visited fortnightly and on holidays, was already being reared by her mother in the country.

Male Respondents

The birth of their first child was most often deliberately delayed by the younger, more educated, and advantaged men without male-dominant views or larger ideal family sizes. In contrast, men with male-dominant views (a woman should risk pregnancy to gain a husband; a story heroine accepts a man's request to have a baby for him) tended not to have used effective contraception prior to the birth of the first child. These men did not regret having many children; they were seemingly sustained by the belief that it is worthwhile to have children regardless of number or ability to care for them.

More than one-third of the first children of male respondents did not live with them or, in the case of visiting unions, their mate. This proportion diminishes sharply with successive children. The kind of crisis that leads to passing on seems most common, as it is for the women, at the birth of the first child. Even these relatively low incidences, however, cannot be compared with those for the women. Most of the men's nonresidential children were from dissolved unions and lived with their mothers, the respondent's former mates. When this is taken into account the proportion of children living with someone other than mother or father decreases sharply, and after the first child it falls to almost nothing.

The Meaning of the First Child

The private and public meanings of her first child for the working-class Jamaican woman arise from her varying levels of self-awareness as an entity separate from others, yet joined with and in some ways moved by them. Her opportunities for autonomous action are limited by the pressures of parent figures, sexual partners, impregnators, and her sense of what is socially needed, expected, and valued. Even the contraceptive-using men in this sample felt that their mates should conform to a cultural expectation of sexual and reproductive submissiveness. But the female respondents said they themselves valued pregnancy as an indicator of their capacity to reproduce and become a mother. Having a baby was not solely or even mainly a response to male needs to demonstrate masculine potency. In this sense, female behavior fits the historically and economically determined tradition that accords high social and personal value to the early demonstration of fertility: the first child is greeted with conscious pride and positive feelings not matched by successive children. Self-awareness emerges with knowledge of one's womanhood primarily through the consummatory experience of delivery. One knows that she is an adult woman less because she is pregnant than because she anticipates that pregnancy will result in a child. Later she experiences the pain of delivery, sees the child, calls for it, cares for it, and expects that someday it—especially a daughter—will care for her.

Another kind of self-awareness anticipates the consequences of behavior before they become inevitable. This is demonstrated in the effective use of contraception by the male respondents, all JFPA clients and, therefore, a special subgroup of concerned Jamaican men. Their awareness allowed them multiple sexual partners and high coital frequency without children. They managed their contraception themselves and did not entrust it to their female partners (table 13). This requires being aware of oneself as an entity capable of autonomous action and free of the constraints of context. Self-awareness is expressed in taking action to interfere with processes previously understood as expected, inevitable, or natural. Such interference is now included within the realm of the "natural." Man's volitional behavior expressing the degree of freedom of which he is capable becomes as natural and acceptable as his conforming to the dictates of other people or of a biology that excludes his mind as a self-regulating apparatus. We assume that the female JFPA clients capable of such

Table 13. Gamma correlations of contraceptive and reproductive performance and attitudes of 283 male JFPA clients.

Factors	Number of children	Effective contraception prior to first child	Reliability of his method choice	Combines M/F methods for reliability	Larger ideal family size	Positive feeling about mate's contraceptive use
Socioeconomic status and modernity						
Education	−.47	.65	.13	.17	−.29	−.02
Occupation	−.26	.40	.12	.26	−.11	.07
Urban birth	−.39	.39	.09	.06	−.26	−.03
Piped water	−.39	.58	.27	.26	−.12	−.04
Literacy	−.26	.40	.27	.18	.03	.13
Mate's education	—	.58	.05	.15	−.29	−.06
Woman should risk pregnancy to get husband	.49	—	.04	−.01	—	.21
Negative attitude toward matriarchy	.45	—	.27	.18	—	−.27
Prefers sons	−.25	—	−.32	−.23	—	−.21
Times moved in Kingston	.36	−.28	.04	.03	.38	−.21
Mate relationship stability						
Relationship stability type	.63	−.43	.42	.34	.84	.30
Previous cohabitors	.53	−.73	−.13	−.23	.30	−.20
Previous visiting relationships	.37	−.25	.14	.11	.32	−.15
Number current visiting relationships	−.24	.39	—	−.02	−.35	—
Supports mother of child	.45	—	.30	.20	—	.29
Feels knows mate well	—	.32	.48	.39	.69	.06
Optimistic about future of relationship	—	−.21	.30	.17	.65	.26

Communication with mate						
Discussed contraception with mate	.39	−.48	—	.48	.56	—
Made joint contraceptive decision	.06	.01	.61	—	.24	.56
Shared mate's contraceptive decision	.02	−.22	—	−.72	−.10	—
Coital history						
Age at first coitus	−.06	—	−.03	.03	—	.15
Frequency of coitus per week	.26	—	.22	.07	—	−.04
Has long periods of abstinence	−.16	—	−.17	−.15	—	−.08
Contraceptive performance/ attitudes						
Effective contraception prior to first child	−.75	1.00	−.14	.09	—	−.06
Large ideal family size	.83	—	.51	.34	1.00	.30
Feels pregnancy controllable	.13	—	.16	.12	—	−.10
Reliable method choice	.26	−.14	1.00	.77	.51	—
Combines male and female methods for reliability	.17	−.09	.77	1.00	.34	.56
Positive feeling about mate's contraceptive use	.11	−.06	—	.56	.30	1.00
Understands reproductive physiology	−.28	.61	.09	—	−.13	−.01
Favors abortion	−.14	.29	.19	—	−.08	.10
Reproductive-paternal performance						
Number of children	1.00	−.75	.26	.17	.83	.11
Wants fewer children	.23	—	−.12	−.27	—	−.13
First child lives with him	.52	—	.29	.26	.69	.25

(continued)

Table 13 continued.

Factors	Number of children	Effective contraception prior to first child	Reliability of his method choice	Combines M/F methods for reliability	Larger ideal family size	Positive feeling about mate's contraceptive use
Attitudes toward women's coping styles in story						
Girl copes independently with pregnancy (aborts)	−.19	—	−.01	.01	—	−.02
Girl copes collaboratively with man's wish for baby	.22	—	.20	.09	—	−.11
Girl copes flexibly with white man's proposal	.05	—	.26	.17	—	−.03
Girl accepts proposal to have baby	.44	—	−.04	−.30	—	−.25

autonomous action, however late or pressed, had an unexpressed awareness of self and self-determination that transcended the self-awareness of their noncontracepting peers.

In the Jamaican working-class setting, the first pregnancy and first child are inevitably the focus of conflicting feelings. Within the family a conflict involves identifications with and prohibitions by the mother or surrogate, who is the primary role model. The repressive rearing of daughters stimulates their resentment and tension by depriving them of sexual-reproductive information and the opportunity for close positive maternal identification. The mother, grandmother, or other surrogate (with whom closeness is even less likely, especially if the child has been passed on) punishes any indication of sexual interest. At the same time, without being consciously recognized as such, she is a model of the kind of behavior she prohibits. These elements contribute to an apprehension in the young girl of the female aspects of her body as disgusting, shameful, or frightening, and symbolic of a forbidden status. Apparent contraceptive passivity and inertia leading to pregnancy, despite the ubiquitous family planning program, reflect denial and dissociation of the devalued body and its reproductive potential from the lived self. They imply as well an unconscious rejection of available knowledge. Such active denial suggests the need to avoid conscious confrontation with a profoundly unacceptable wish. One such wish might be to displace the mother from her role as the central reproductively capable female in the household. The process of pregnancy, then, acquires a symptomatic reconstitutive function: the girl unconsciously displaces her mother as she revalues her body by affirming its child-producing capability. Another unconscious wish might be to escape the female role entirely to the degree that it involves relating sexually and submissively to Jamaican men. This wish would accord with the existence of a basically adversary relationship between the Jamaican woman and men, suggested earlier. She tends to see them as economically but not affectively valuable, and not, in most instances, as the prime object of her responsibility. She has usually had to undo her mother's prohibitions without an intimate and consistent mate. The high frequency of noncommunication with and nonsupport from the father of her first child contributes to the reconstitutive function of initial pregnancy and childbirth. Her previously devalued reproductive potential becomes realized less through a sustained, emotionally supportive partnership than through her own private efforts.

Female respondents expressed conscious resentment toward both their depriving mothers and their unreliable first impregnators. In no instance was this resentment directed against the first child. One-fourth gave neutral or indifferent responses toward the first child and expressed negative feelings about giving birth. It is plausible that negative feelings about the birth indicate negative feelings at some hidden level about the baby as well. Given the high frequency of negative interaction with the baby's father, the question arises whether there exist masked destructive or hostile feelings toward the baby as the unrecognized embodiment of the man who helped create it. The resolution of unconscious conflict between the wish to keep and care for the child and the desire symbolically to sever the ties with its father or take revenge upon him is facilitated by yet other cultural forms. Passing the child on to be reared by others and harsh child-rearing practices permit the expression of destructive wishes aimed against its father without requiring conscious confrontation of those wishes. In any event, successive male partners are not enthusiastic about supporting children from a former union. The characteristics of the passing-on respondents somewhat resemble Brodber's generalizations about child abandoners. These are likely to be mothers under 26 years old with less than two children: "Rather than being destitute, it seems probable that disappointment with the response of the preferred source of help, the baby's father, produces a sort of apathy toward making alternative arrangements, a state of mind, which if allowed to persist, predisposes mothers toward relegating the problem of the child to be cared for out of existence" (1974, pp. 23-24). Especially in the case of young women who have migrated into Kingston from rural areas, often establishing a sexual union for the first time, isolation even from the informal sanctions of the kin group is common.

When the man departs with the onset of pregnancy or around the time of delivery, the only person to give social meaning to the child's existence is the new mother. If she does not feel competent or willing to do this she may be inclined to give it away to be reared by someone else.

The personal significance of passing on may be more intense for young women who were themselves passed on to be reared by surrogates. Indeed, as already noted, passing on one's child is correlated with having been reared by grandmother. In no instance, however, despite hints and occasional direct expressions of resentment at having been given away for rearing, did one of the passing-on respondents recognize that she was doing to her child what had been done to her. The accepted cultural pattern permits (without recognition) disposition of the conceptus, sometimes the product of intercourse as a disguised act of rebellion against one's mother, to another person. The final phase of this symptomatic sequence for the ambivalent woman would be either employment of the flexible opportunities for visiting her passed-on child or ensuring its complete disappearance from her everyday reality. The degree to which this disappearance is hindered by her persistent memories or feelings or by a continued need to disavow the child's existence is determined by early biographical as much as contextual factors.

Passing on may be a successful way of dealing with the unacceptable vectors of conflict and their associated tensions. In this case it may be viewed as a move toward a new identity. If it helps the woman gain a new job and/or a new mate—and in any case survive—it may also be viewed as adaptive.

Another, often unconscious, source of conflict is the matrifocal-matricentric household. In this setting social constraints on the floating male are minimal. Inexperienced females, uninformed and frustrated by maternal restrictions and unprotected by older male relatives, are easily available to him. These factors increase the likelihood that as the man proves himself sexually effective by producing a first or successive pregnancy, for himself, he will disappear leaving the young woman to be absorbed, now as another adult female with child, into the matricentric household. If she wishes, the first child, having fulfilled its function as a symbol of her own fertility, can be turned over to her mother for rearing or, when a new man enters her life, passed on to one of its father's relatives. The child's significance as the catalyzing nucleus of a new family is minimal compared to its instrumental and expressive meanings for the mother alone.

In summary, in this context early pregnancy and the appearance of her first child, preceded by early first coitus without contraception, appear to have a variety of meanings for the Jamaican working-class woman. Most prominently these are concerned with ambivalent identification with mother, adversary relationships with male partners, and the primary significance of her own body in the production of the first child. Pregnancy is an introduction to the woman's assumption of the parenting role of both sexes. She learns that having a baby "for" her man does not ensure his permanence. This is the time when he leaves her for another woman who will "give him" his next baby. His departure leaves her to be a father as well as mother to her new child (Clarke, 1957). This socially imposed necessity to "father" as well as to "mother" the new baby may contribute to a fantasied gratification of a particular variant of the wish to escape the traditional female role, an unconscious wish to reproduce without the participation of the male, perhaps in a sense of a "drive to become both sexes" (Kubie, 1974): she has produced the new child single-handed. The individual private and unconscious significance of the act is made more plausible because it can be masked. The repression of its meaning is aided by the fact that it conforms to the public patterns of early pregnancy and child rearing without the consistent aid and companionship of a male partner in a female-dominated context.

The woman's perception of the infant as a private function of her own body, a demonstration of personal capacity for which no one else is responsible, was most graphically expressed by psychiatric patients. A 28-year-old unmarried domestic, already the mother of one, said when she learned of her pregnancy, "All one have to do is touch me and I make a baby . . . One little sex and I get pregnant . . . Some people die just to have one." She did not tell the "baby-father" because "I wasn't friends with him . . . just had a little piece with him . . . no need to tell him" (Brody, 1974).

Early first coitus, first union, and first pregnancy, associated with adherence to traditional matrifocal-matricentric beliefs, reaffirm the significance of having children as a primarily female activity. They diminish the importance of a collaborative relationship with a partner with whom one might negotiate or at least share feelings and ideas about contracepting and reproducing. Early first pregnancy also fits the maternal tradition by repeating the mother's behavior, conforming to what might be called a "culture of motherhood" in the sense of a socially inherited design for living (Kluckhohn, 1944). The complex beliefs involved in this socially inherited design include the expectation that one's mother will care for the first baby. It develops in a context characterized by seeming paradoxes. The mothers of the most matricentric women tend to have exercised repressive control over their behavior, refused sexual information, and threatened explusion with early pregnancy; yet they themselves had had early, unmarried, and frequent pregnancies. Our respondents referred regularly to their mother's anger at their first pregnancies, but none seemed to doubt her willingness to care for the babies.

The experienced sequence from coitus through pregnancy to delivery reflects the psychological activities of both disavowal and reversal. In the first, denial and repression aided by the existence of particular cultural patterns facilitate ignoring the reproductive consequences of intercourse and the disguised expression of unacceptable wishes through these consequences. In the second, positive self-affirmation takes place, undoing the passive status into which the girl was forced by her mother, males, and society in general. She utilizes intercourse and first conception as an active experience of mastery, revaluing her body and affirming its reproductive competence, symbolizing her dependence upon no one but herself. At the broadest sociocultural level the conflict is between the impulses to achieve personal freedom (regulating one's own fertility like other bodily and mental processes) and to conform to the pressure of pronatal values.

8 Sexual Partnerships, Marriage, and Reproductive Behavior

> Maybe the younger girl is friendly with the older woman's husband and she has come to fight her.
>
> *Female respondent's description*
> *of a TAT card*

> Jamaican women have enough opportunities if they want to make use of men.
>
> *A female respondent*

Legal marriage, often termed "lawful" or "Christian," comes late for those Jamaican women who achieve it at all. Approximately one-third of all women of reproductive age (15 to 44) islandwide have, according to the most recently available census figures (table 14), never had a partnership sufficiently durable to be regarded as a "union." Of Kingston Parish women in this age range, encompassing all social classes, only 10.2 percent were legally married. By age 45 to 64, however, 31.5 percent were married.

The first relationships are with men who father one (or in some cases all) of their children. These early sexual unions, as a rule, are part-time. Our data and those from the public maternity hospital in Kingston (table 14) indicate that the large majority of Jamaican women at the time of their first or second pregnancy are neither legally married nor cohabiting.

The special nature of this culture in terms of the social sanctions applied to reproduction is indicated by a comparison with

Table 14. Union status of Jamaican women, in percentages.

Union status	150 study subjects, 1974-1975[a]	197 Victoria Jubilee Hospital confinements, October–December 1969[b]	National census, 1960[c]
Visiting	43.3	46.6	34.9
Common-law, cohabiting	34.0 } 48.7	46.6 } 50.6	19.2 } 46.0
Legally married, cohabiting	14.7	4.0	26.8
Cohabiting with or visiting man other than common-law or legal mate	6.7 } 8.0	— } 2.8	— } 19.8
Temporarily no regular mate	1.3	2.8	—

a. For women aged 16-47, 17.3 percent of current relationships were of one year or less and 18.7 percent had lasted one to two years in duration. Twenty-two relationships (14.7 percent) had been broken because of the mate's emigration.

b. Data on women aged 15-40 + from E. Brodber, *Abandonment of children in Jamaica* (Mona, Jamaica: Institute of Social and Economic Research, University of the West Indies, 1974), p. 11.

c. Data from E. Brodber, *Abandonment of children in Jamaica*, p. 18.

United States figures. Although approximately 60 percent of first births to U.S. white teenagers and 90 percent to black teenagers between 1975-1978 were premaritally conceived, more than 58 percent of the pregnant white group and 8 percent of the pregnant black group were married prior to delivery. Just four years earlier, in 1971-1974, the marriage rate for premaritally pregnant U.S. teenagers was higher: nearly 65 percent for whites and over 17 percent for blacks.

By age 20-24 the rate of premaritally conceived births for U.S. white women between 1975-1978 was much lower, only 17 percent, and for blacks 56 percent. For these whites postpregnancy marriage occurred at about the same rate as for younger women (58.4 percent) but for blacks it was much higher (27.3 percent), suggesting the increased value accorded to marital status with increasing age (O'Connell and Moore, 1980).

The Jamaican girl, in contrast to her U.S. white counterpart, and to a lesser degree to her black counterpart, tends to remain in her mother's home even with her second or later pregnancy. Still adolescent, she continues to be "visited" there by her man, and rears their child(ren). Marriage during pregnancy is rare. The young woman remains a daughter, unmarried, emotionally and materially dependent and socially subordinate, as she gradually assumes the role of mother. Although her own mother has accused her of wanting to become a "big woman" through intercourse and childbearing, she does not in fact achieve this status so long as she remains in the parental home. In time—the age range is variable—she may move out to a tenement room, especially if she has left the country to find work in Kingston. She may acquire a yard of her own. Or she and her former visiting partner, or a new one, may decide to share a dwelling in a common-law marriage. This can have the force and value for many couples of a legal marriage, of which it is often the precursor, but it does not provide the security or social status of the latter.

In these circumstances it is plausible to regard unstable conjugal relations as a salient feature of the lives of Jamaican women of childbearing and child-rearing age. An aspect of this instability is poor communication between members of the conjugal pair, often involving deliberate concealment by one or both of important feelings, attitudes, and activities from the other. This lack of communication can have profound consequences for a joint activity such as contraception and planning the number and spacing of pregnancies.

The Historical Roots of Jamaican Family Structure

The nature of the relationship between the sexes in Jamaica has been attributed to a series of interrelated factors. These include insufficient employment, the frequent movement of men in search of work, the external migration of both sexes for the same reason, and the low status of women. Although there is ample room for disagreement, a considerable literature also suggests its roots in African residuals and in Jamaica's colonial history, especially the condition of slavery. The English colonial government, concentrating on the production of sugarcane on large estates, began to import large numbers of Africans to the island in the 1660s. By the mid-eighteenth century, Jamaicans of African descent outnumbered European inhabitants by estimates ranging from 7 to 1, to 15 to 1 (JIS, 1972; Norris, 1962; Black, 1973). European men, accompanied by relatively few of their women, mixed freely with the female slaves and soon produced a growing mulatto class. By the time the trade was legally abolished in 1808 these Afro-Europeans greatly outnumbered the Europeans. Though usually freed and sometimes educated by their fathers, they had few privileges or civil rights as members of a third legal caste (the other two being free whites and black slaves). Not allowed to own significant amounts of property and wishing to avoid manual agricultural labor—the mark of slavery—they congregated in towns and became clerks, small businessmen, and tradesmen. Their difference from the untaught black Africans and their descendents was further intensified by heavy slave importation in the last years of the trade: 63,045 came into Jamaica in 1801-1807. A majority of these last arrivals remained on the plantations, left to educate their own children. Gradually, however, through a process of cumulative adaptation and amalgamation of African cultures, a new pattern developed tending to emphasize elements common to all groups. By the 1830s an "Afro-Jamaican culture" had been solidly established (Curtin, 1955).

These factors added racial overtones to political and economic differences between town and country. Even in the mid-twentieth century prominence and prestige, wealth and power continued to be "distributed in terms of light pigmentation" (M. G. Smith, 1960, p. 38), associated with urban rather than rural residence. A recent novel of Kingston life describes "the housewives with their brown and olive-skinned legs . . . and their gardener boys with their black torsos . . . From the lumpiness of her features and her unstraightened hair you could tell that she was recently from the country" (Patterson, 1971, pp. 126-127).

The urban-rural distinction, of course, was never absolute and became progressively less so in the mid-twentieth century with increasing movement from the country into the Kingston area. But town employment opportunities were always few and men earned an intermittent living, "scuffing" about, spending much time in idleness, and depending upon relatives for sustenance. The value of a large family upon whom one could depend in time of need was taken for granted.

In contrast to this townward movement, some of the black ex-slaves remained on the great estates after emancipation as wage workers, eventually buying small pieces of land from the owners. Most—perhaps more independent—moved to the unoccupied hills, sometimes still designated "the mountain," where they created their own villages and farming communities. Some simply squatted on Crown lands. In this way a rural black peasantry gradually emerged as a definable class. For them the value of children as field hands and as helpers with farm chores was unquestioned.

The availability of unused land to anyone who could cultivate it may have reinforced the feeling that large families would always have space into which to expand. It may have also supported the value of internal migration as a problem-solving maneuver. Family land tenure, found in much of the rural population of Jamaica and elsewhere in the Caribbean, could contribute to a matriarchal, matrifocal family organization to the degree that it supported female dominance, with nonlandowning males coming to live on the woman's land—according to Clarke (1953, 1957), a West African vestige reflecting the shortage of land in both Africa and Jamaica. In an agricultural society with few economic alternatives, siblings who have inherited the land as a group may remain together at the expense of conjugal ties.

Nonlegalized cohabiting or "visiting" conjugal unions in which families center about a mother and her children, often with a grandmother and sometimes with other female relatives, are regarded by some observers as African residuals, the heritage of slavery, adaptations to current socioeconomic conditions, or functions of all three. Herskovits (1946, 1948) is a major exponent of the idea that the New World domestic system is based mainly on West Africa, where the family pattern was frequently polygamous, with separate households for each wife and her children.

According to Curtin's account (1955) of island life between

1830 and 1865 and Norris's essay on Jamaican identity (1962), the Jamaican male slave usually had a long-term domestic partner, perhaps more than one, who with children constituted a social unit. The owners, however, apparently discouraged long-term or at least monogamous relations, believing that frequent changes of partners made the women more fertile. They themselves were models of promiscuity and high fertility. In the absence of a white wife, a "housekeeping" arrangement would be made with a brown woman—which she considered more desirable than marriage with a man of her own class. Maidservants were also concubines and were given the privilege of less work and better treatment. For brown men this added sexual competition to the sources of racial animosity.

A more forceful summary, revealing the attitude of a contemporary Jamaican social scientist, states: "This was a society . . . in which the institution of marriage was officially condemned among both masters and slaves; in which the family was unthinkable to the vast majority of the population and promiscuity the norm" (Patterson, 1973, p. 9). Although the breakdown of sexual mores was general among blacks transported to the New World, "in no other area was the degree of sexual abandonment so great as in Jamaica . . . [due to] the similar breakdown of such mores among the dominant white group" (p. 159).

There is general agreement that the conditions of slavery made it virtually impossible for the average black male to maintain an effective role as a family head or father: he could not assert himself economically, nor could he protect his female partners from sexual domination by whites or browns. Brown women were described as intensely contemptuous not only of black men but also of men of their own color (Patterson, 1973). Even after middle age, when stable relationships were more frequent, the man's familial authority was minimal because his partner's children were by other men and his own would be living with his previous mates.

Patterson's review of early sources notes as causes of high fecundity the polygamous mating patterns of the more prosperous slaves, the positive attitudes of African-born women to childbearing and child care, and the fact that most were brought to the islands between the ages of 15 and 25. On the other hand, many factors, among them the effects of heavy plantation labor, an extremely high infant mortality, and the marked excess of males over females, acted to control population growth. Moreover, a considerable number of slave women apparently did not want to produce children doomed to lives of servitude and punishment. Abortion seems to have been widely practiced. Venereal disease was common. And as new generations appeared young Creole women began to control their childbearing, feeling that it reduced their attractiveness to white males.

By the time the missionaries arrived, Jamaican women tended to regard Christian marriage as a mark of subordination to the male. The missionaries, however, attacked concubinage as well as drumming, dancing, and other Afro-Jamaican customs. They were strict in respect to marriage and discouraged the baptism of illegitimate children. Although this barred the majority of the population from the church, Jamaicans would not get married and public opinion did not condemn concubinage. In 1938 a royal commission was appointed to investigate the "disorganization" of family life and the "social, moral and economic evils of promiscuity" (WIRC Report, 1945, p. 424, cited by M. G. Smith, 1966). In 1944-1945 the commission initiated a "Mass Marriage Movement." The effect of this, however, was minimal and short-lived, for it was "based on the erroneous notion that because the elite and lower class employed a single word, marriage, to denote a particular conjugal institution, this had identical or very similar meanings, value and significance" for both social strata (M. G. Smith, 1966).

Current Attitudes of Women toward Men and Marriage

The personal meaning of the conjugal relationship for Jamaican women today is suggested by the tendency of our 150 respondents to feel negative about men (70 percent), to regard them instrumentally, and to value their partners less than their mothers (56 percent). Most respondents regarded Jamaican men as "all alike." Although they defined the major male role as that of economic provider (88 percent), less than half regarded men as having higher status than women. Approximately one-third recognized a possible fathering role for their partners, but only half believed that having children without marriage is bad, and none specified companionship as a conjugal function. Informal conversation made it clear, however, that they counted on their mates to take them (and sometimes their children) to bars, movies, dances, sports, the beach, or private social gatherings. When this did not occur it was a source of considerable dissatisfaction and friction. It also figured, along with a decrease in the frequency of sexual intercourse, in the woman's suspicion that her man might be seeing someone else.

Working-class Jamaican women are as jealous, angry, and disappointed as people elsewhere when their mates form alliances with new partners. Their matricentric orientation does not protect them from pain and feelings of loss or rejection. Apparent tolerance of male infidelity and failure to support their children has been regarded as an indication of low self-esteem. It may more immediately reflect, however, the man's absolute lack of economic resources and the woman's realistically minimal expectations of support and constancy. Middle-class women urging abandoned young mothers to seek redress in the courts tend to be met with the response, "If me do that, him never come back and we never get nothin."

Despite jealousy, anger, and interest in the mate as a social escort and source of economic support, his personal significance is devalued. Fewer than half the women felt a primary responsibility to him. The majority placed higher value on the enduring relationship with their mother, however ambivalently they had described her, and they were evidently prepared to sacrifice some aspects of the conjugal relationship in order to preserve it. The mother appeared to symbolize the female in general. The sense of belonging to a dominant female group was often expressed directly: "A woman can get anything quicker than a man." Or "men are so much a failure these days." Or "I don't know what will happen between me and my [common-law] husband. My mother comes first. I look for it from my children too."

In many more cases, identification with the female group was implied in the negative evaluation of men who leave the women to do the essential work of child rearing and transmitting family values: "the men don't like to take care of family." Or "They have children all around." Or "They don't love married life." Or, as one unmarried woman in her late twenties, already the mother of five, put it: "They just don't care what want to happen to you . . . Just having children, then leave them . . . They don't conscious."

Many expressed a preference to remain unmarried, fearing they would be trapped in a relationship that would eventually prove burdensome. Some, upon finding themselves pregnant, refused offers to cohabit because "he still keep a lot of girls." Their mothers had often counseled against permanent attachments under these circumstances. These attitudes do not seem solely consequences of personal experience but also part of a socially inherited complex of values and beliefs about the centrality of mothers.

The Current Sexual Partnership

Feelings and Attitudes

Less than one-third of the 127 unmarried members (84.7 percent) of the sample expected legalization of their current union. Only 60 percent of the entire group received major financial support from their current mate. About half the total, though not especially happy about their unions, looked forward to a degree of stability; that is, they did not expect a major change in the status of the relationship. The others were almost equally divided between expectations of improvement or deterioration.

Just under half the women, including the small proportion who were legally married, lived together with their sexual partners (table 14). Conjugal stability increases with age: an insignificant correlation between age and the duration of the first conjugal union increases to more substantial levels for the second (gamma

.31) and third (gamma .43). Women who are older at the onset of their later unions are apt to remain with the same mate for longer periods of time. The likelihood that a couple will live together rather than visit each other also increases with age (gamma .30). There is no significant correlation, however, between living together and feeling emotionally satisfied with the current mate. On the contrary, the older the woman, the longer the cohabiting relationship, and the higher the reproductive performance, the more likely she was to report (gamma .28) feeling that men are irresponsible. There was a high degree of conjugal dissatisfaction and little sense of an intimate, affectively reciprocal, mutually supporting relationship between mates, even between those who share the same dwelling. These working-class women do not relate to more economically substantial partners as the years pass. Nor can they count with the passage of time on receiving financial support from their current mate, discussion or agreement with him about contraceptive use, emotional satisfaction from the relationship, or positive expectations for its future. In short, while there is a greater tendency for women to cohabit rather than visit as they grow older, and for longer periods of time, the conjugal relationship promises neither economic nor emotional security. They do not regard it as having more of a future than the younger women do their current relationships. Several replied, when asked about their expectations, "Nothing." The most frequent response was simply "I don't know." When questioned about their reasons for remaining with their current mate, most began by saying that they didn't know what else to do, and many revealed fantasies that either she or he would soon depart. Typical replies about the man's attitude were "I'm not getting it" or "Women have it hard, men give nothing for the pickney" or "I feel like I'm talking, but he not hearing." One woman put it bluntly: "No use me talkin' . . . Him too ignorant." In contrast, a man who came back regularly from working in Cuba and with whom the respondent was discussing marriage she called "a steady man."

It seems likely that many older and more experienced women who have been through several visiting phases and now share a dwelling with their mates may share more family responsibilities with them, communicate more, and therefore engage them in a more egalitarian manner. They often derive some self-esteem from the social status of being part of a known union. Furthermore, despite the lack of certain economic help they can usually count on occasional money, food, clothing, or gifts from their mates for themselves or their children. These women are not clearly positive or negative, but ambivalent about their mates and conjugal situations.

Visiting

The most prevalent union type (43.3 percent of the sample) is a visiting one. The man usually comes on a regular basis to the woman's home for purposes of sexual intercourse, child rearing, and arranging for economic support or companionship. Those who attend church often do so as a couple as they might if cohabiting or legally married. Visiting frequency varies considerably over time, especially in unions of long duration. Changes are usually the result of the man's retreat "to the country" to work, with the expectation that he will eventually move back to Kingston or that the respondent will sooner or later join him. Under these circumstances sexual intercourse may be limited to weekends and occasionally less often. Such moves sometimes stimulate fear that the union is coming to an end. Relatively infrequent visits also occur when a country woman moves to the city leaving her mate behind with the expectation that he will eventually find a job enabling him to join her.

When younger women live in the parental home the opportunity for sexual relations may be constrained by lack of privacy or by friction between the man and her family. Others, migrant into the city, live alone, with their children, or with female relatives or friends. Those who live alone are most apt to see their visiting partners frequently. Between one-fourth and one-third of the visiting couples saw each other almost every evening or in nonworking hours, usually for two or three hours at a time (although they did not have intercourse each time). There may also be longer visits during weekends and holidays. When the woman lives alone, her mate often spends the entire night with her, especially on weekends. When she lives with her parents he may stay in her room or occasionally she in his. Lack of space and privacy requires the couple to engage in sexual intercourse outdoors, in the man's room, in hotels, or in the home of a friend.

About three-fourths of the women who lived separately occasionally visit their partner's dwelling. Many, however, complained that their man did not wish them to do so, probably because he kept another woman. In some instances these visits occurred in pursuit of promised but unmaterialized economic support for the children, and in some simply because more than the expected time had elapsed since the last meeting. An unexpected visit may result in screaming accusations and a fight. Several respondents acknowledged, usually with feeling, that part of their mate's time and money was regularly devoted to another household: "Him have a girl near where he used to work and she had a baby for him, so he not here so much."

Women who only visited with their partners were not socioeconomically different from those who lived together. Their initiation into the sexual-reproductive career, however, was different in their having had a less satisfying experience with the man who made them first pregnant. Only 27 percent, in contrast with 45 percent of the cohabiting women, still maintained their union with the man with whom they had had their first child. Whereas the majority of women in the sample were separated from their first impregnator, those in a visiting relationship at the time of the research interview had suffered more life disruption in this regard than those who cohabited and thus had a more stable current support system. Some women, of course, were already married or cohabiting at the time of first pregnancy. In these relatively few instances the child had been planned or prepared for and at least socially anticipated. Most women separated from their mates prior to delivery or during the child's very early years went on to find another visiting mate, but some persisting unions moved from visiting to cohabiting status.

Cohabiting

Approximately one-third of the respondents, a few of whom had previously been visiting, were in a common-law relationship, sharing a dwelling with their mate. Including the approximately 15 percent who were legally married, almost half were currently living together. A few (6.7 percent) maintained primary relationships with men other than those with whom they lived; they had occasional sex with their common-law or legal mate, but described more frequent and emotionally involving contact with someone else, whom they would "visit." (These are regarded for statistical purposes as cohabiting.) Only two of the 150 women (both legally separated from their husbands) had no regular mate at the time of the interview but had sufficiently frequent sexual intercourse to make them decide to maintain their contraceptive status.

Duration

Almost one-fifth of the current unions of the 150 respondents had begun in the year preceding the interview (table 14); almost half were of three years or less; and only one-fourth had persisted for seven years or more.

The brief duration of many early sexual partnerships reflects the casual way in which they were initiated. For example, a 30-year-old woman recalled that at age 14 she was at a boy's home: "We were just playing and it happen." They continued to have intercourse at approximately weekly intervals for about three months and "then we stopped talking to each other." In sharp contrast, this woman's second sexual partner was her current mate, with whom she had been living for 12 years with no plans for marriage. In approximately three-fourths of the disrupted unions, the man simply deserted. Approximately 15 percent of the women reported unions broken because of the man's emigration to the United States, Canada, or England. When she herself had severed the relationship it was usually because she had discovered that he had another woman. For example, "I was pregnant for him and he went back to live with another woman who had already had two babies for him." In several instances she left because of disagreements with his female relatives: "He had a nasty mother" or "I got vexed with his grandmother." The woman's own mother was also cited several times as a reason for disrupting the relationship. For example, "She said I was too small for those things." In a few instances the father was the crucial factor. One woman was engaged but her father objected to the proposed marriage. She therefore established a common-law relationship with her mate and had "a son for him." Then, after three years, the man moved to New York, where he had a job, and she lived alone, supporting her child, with little expectation of reunion or marriage.

Current Household Arrangements

It was difficult to determine exactly who was the most influential voice in each dwelling occupied by a female respondent and it is probably fair to conclude that the actual division of household heads between the sexes was approximately even. The leading role was usually attributed to the person who owned the house, had lived in it longest, paid most of the rent, or coordinated domestic tasks and resolved quarrels. When a viable older male relative was present he tended to be so designated. When a grandmother but no older male was present, she was so viewed and sometimes given money for household expenses by younger employed persons.

The largest proportion, almost one-third of the respondents, shared their dwelling with a common-law partner, most often referred to as a "boy friend." Her children by him (and occasionally hers and, rarely, his by a former mate) were usually there, and in a few cases other relatives as well. In some instances she and her mate had the dwelling to themselves. Another 21 women lived with their legal husbands and usually other family members as well, for a total of almost half who were cohabiting; all of these women had had at least one child.

Sixty women lived without men, either alone or with their children or in exclusively female households. Thirty of these, 19 with their children, had no adult companions, male or female. In general, noncohabiting women tended to band together with others, usually sisters or maternal relatives, to form households; when the households included men other than fathers they, too, were apt to be maternal relatives.

Partner Diversity and Reproductive Behavior

The current conjugal status of these women and the nature of their domestic arrangements must be understood in the context of a career of multiple sexual and reproductive partnerships with minimal communication about reproductive matters. Only 57 percent of those having a second pregnancy, for example, had been impregnated by the same man who produced their first, and the number of partners increased with the number of pregnancies. Of 61 women with a fourth pregnancy, just over one-fourth had been produced by the first impregnator and 16.3 percent were the consequence of coitus with a fourth man (table 15). Although sex and reproduction appear to have been the major concern of successive conjugal unions, fewer than two-thirds of the 150 women had discussed contraception with their current mate, and for these mutual agreement about its use was not universal. A significant proportion (one-fifth) made the decision by themselves without discussion. In these instances they did not tell their mates until they had already obtained and were employing the methods or the mates discovered it themselves. The women who made contraceptive decisions unilaterally tended to be those who, having had several previous partners, still lived alone and had a visiting relationship with their current sexual partner. Their earlier experiences had led them to distrust men and feel that they must assume responsibility for their own welfare (Brody, Ottey, and LaGranade, 1976). A 25-year-old unmarried mother of six voiced an attitude implied by many: "The main thing that holds women down in Jamaica is that the men don't give a chance to get teachment about birth control. Man wants to keep a woman down in the house all the time."

An index of partner diversity is the number of impregnators per pregnancy for women who have been pregnant more than

Table 15. Relationship of successive pregnancies of 133 Jamaican women to impregnators.

Pregnancy number	Number of women pregnant	By male 1	By male 2	By male 3	By male 4	By male 5	By male 6
1	133	100.0%	0.0%	0.0%	0.0%	0.0%	0.0%
2	102	56.9	43.1	0.0	0.0	0.0	0.0
3	78	37.1	37.1	25.8	0.0	0.0	0.0
4	61	26.2	34.5	23.0	16.3	0.0	0.0
5	40	22.5	27.5	22.5	20.0	7.5	0.0
6	22	18.2	13.6	18.2	31.9	13.6	4.5

once. The variation among respondents is largely accounted for by the number of visiting mates reported by a woman per unit time of her sexually active career prior to the research interview. That is, the likelihood of a woman's having been pregnant more often than the median for her age group was higher if she had had multiple visiting mates. She tended to have become pregnant in consequence of each visiting union—to "have a baby for" each of her regular sexual partners. Thus, a series of visiting partners produced more babies than a single, long-term, cohabiting relationship. Census data do in fact show that more women in visiting unions than those cohabiting or married have three or more children. Fewer in the visiting category have none (table 16). Within the total legally unmarried group the residual variation in number of impregnators among women with more than one pregnancy is probably accounted for by their having actually shared a dwelling with several boy friends, in contrast with simply visiting.

Some corollaries of high partner diversity appear to precede and others to follow having had several mates. Less educated women with more traditional matricentric beliefs, having had little open communication with their mothers about sex and early and unsatisfactory initiations into their coital-reproductive careers, tended to have had sexual relations with and been impregnated by larger numbers of men. Women who had had many mates and impregnators expressed negative feelings about being pregnant, did not agree that a story heroine should accept a white man's offer to support her in return for sex, and felt negative about having a large family. They had experienced fetal loss and had passed on children to be reared by someone else. A working-class Jamaican woman who had had two pregnancies by different men had already experienced the emotional, physical, and economic impact of child care under adverse circumstances. Nevertheless, she was unlikely to discuss contraception or to ask for and receive financial support from later mates, for whom she would have additional babies.

As noted in chapter 5, more than one-third of the 17 women who had never been pregnant had already had two regular visit-

Table 16. Number and percentage of children according to union status of Jamaican women not attending school, by age.

Union type	Age 20-24				Age 30-34				Age 40-44			
	N	0 children	%	3+ children	%	N	0 children	%	3+ children	%	N	0 children	%	3+ children	%
Married	7,438	1,329	17.7	2,269	30.5	16,527	1,136	6.9	11,655	62.4	20,480	1,942	9.5	14,691	71.7
Common-law	18,681	1,864	10.0	7,918	42.4	13,429	912	6.7	10,276	76.5	8,463	992	11.7	5,747	67.9
Visiting	7,596	0	0.0	2,822	37.1	1,572	0	0.0	1,373	87.3	354	0	0.0	325	91.8

Source: *1970 Population census of the Commonwealth Caribbean; vol. 8, Fertility* (Kingston: Census Research Programme, University of the West Indies, 1976), p. 10.

ing mates; three had had prolonged periods of celibacy, one for 11 years; five had come to the clinic seeking contraceptives at their current mate's request; two had decided to contracept without telling their mates; in only one case could the decision be described as joint.

Male Respondents

Union Status

Like the women, the largest proportion of the 283 men (40.1 percent) were in visiting unions. Their more advantaged socioeconomic status, however, was indicated by the fact that more than one-third were legally married and most of these lived with their wives. Another one-fourth shared dwellings with common-law mates, for a total of 58.8 percent currently cohabiting. Age was also more significant for the men than the women. When those under age 23 are eliminated, almost three-fourths lived with their primary partners. Only a few (1.1 percent) said their sexual relations were limited to pickups.

The union situation of the males is more complicated than that of the females because of their acknowledged multiplicity of current mates. Very few limited their sexual partnerships (with regular, expectable visits and shared social, economic, and affectional as well as sexual relations) to one woman (table 17). Most of those living with a primary partner acknowledged at least one additional regular visiting mate; of those with primary visiting unions more than two-thirds visited with two or more women. More than one-fourth of all the men reported that they were engaging simultaneously in three or more unions. Nonetheless, they granted special status to their primary partner. Almost all stated that they talked with her about their future lives together and over three-fourths were optimistic about a lasting union. Two-thirds also claimed they supplied her major economic support. Over half in visiting unions reported 16 to 30 visits monthly to their primary mate. Only two-thirds, however, felt they knew their mate "well," and only 29 percent knew her "very" well.

Table 17. Number of current sexual unions of 283 male JFPA clients, in percentages.

Current partner type	None	One	Two	Three or more
Visiting or cohabiting, total	1.1[a]	28.0	44.0	26.9
Visiting, total	13.8	44.7	32.3	9.2
Secondary visiting (primary cohabiting)	12.7[a]	16.7	11.7	17.7[b]
Primary visiting	59.9[c]	15.8	15.8	8.8[d]

Note: Of clients ages 15-57, 58.8 percent are currently cohabiting; of the 228 over age 23, 73.2 percent are currently cohabiting.

a. 1.1 percent have casual partners only; 12.7 percent who cohabit have no visiting mates in addition.

b. 78 percent of cohabitors have 1 or more regular visiting mates.

c. 5.3 percent of cohabitors have no visiting mates but pick up women for occasional sex.

d. 69 percent of men whose primary unions are visiting, visit with 2 or more women.

Most (71.1 percent) reported having had two or more visiting relationships prior to the current one, but only 16 percent had had previous cohabitors.

Another 15.8 percent of the men lived with one or both parents, and 12.8 percent resided in dwellings headed by siblings or other relatives. A considerably smaller proportion than the women, 9.8 percent, lived alone; the remaining 1.8 percent were with persons or families to whom they were not related.

Among the 228 men aged 23 and over, those who lived with their sexual partner, in contrast with those who only visited, were likely to talk with her about contraception (gamma .85), although they did not necessarily agree that she should contracept. They also were likely, however, to embrace traditional male-dominance values. These men tended to have a higher ideal family size (gamma .92) and to define women as submissive to male desires for children. (This is indicated by their interpretation of a story situation, their feeling that women should risk pregnancy to gain marriage (gamma .60), and the fact that they did not report

negative feelings about having children without being married.)
They also believed in the traditional familial child-caring role of
the grandmother.

Other indicators of a conservative viewpoint and high value
placed on reproductive performance include negative correlations between cohabiting status and having contracepted prior to
the first child (gamma $-.66$), currently combining male and female methods for greater contraceptive security (gamma $-.57$),
and favoring abortion (gamma $-.34$).

Unlike the situation for working-class women reflected in both
the sample and the national census figures, cohabiting status for
these men is associated with having produced a larger overall
number of children and with having produced more than the
median for the age group. Within this relatively well-educated,
high-status sample of male contraceptive users, the current cohabitors tended to be less educated, with less educated mates,
less often of urban birth, and of lower occupational status than
the noncohabitors. Thus, the larger number of children may be
less a function of living together than of the lower socioeconomic
status and more traditional beliefs of those who cohabit.

Partner Diversity

Despite their multiple mating, the frequency of multiple impregnation is less for these males than for working-class women.
Approximately 28 percent of the men having a second child had
had it with a woman other than the mother of their first (compared with 43 percent of the women having their second baby by
a second father). In even sharper contrast with the women, less
than one-third of their first children were born to women with
whom they were in a visiting union at the time. The remainder
were married or common-law cohabiting in almost equal numbers. Almost half the mothers of these first children still cohabited with the respondent at the time of the research interview,
and even more respondents tended to be cohabiting with or married to the mothers of their second and subsequent children.
Thus, the successively impregnated partners of these men repre-

sent a movement toward conjugal stability rather than a simple series of visiting unions.

The apparent value placed by the cohabiting men on male dominance and fertility is not associated with their having impregnated several females. In fact, having a different mother for each of two children is correlated with a wish for fewer children (gamma .86) and a smaller ideal family size (gamma .51). These condom-using men have in general made an early decision to regulate their fertility, and they produce their children with one, or at least fewer, mates than the others. It is possible that deliberate concern with separating sexual from reproductive activity is associated with less need to affirm masculine status through impregnating many women, and thus with the capacity for more responsible parenthood.

The *total* number of mates to date for each respondent compared with others of the same age group is not significantly correlated with his socioeconomic status. The men who had had more sexual partners had begun their coital careers early (gamma .52) and thus had had a longer period of habituated sexual exposure. This is part of a cluster including a high current frequency of sexual intercourse (gamma .53), valuing female submission to a man's wish for a baby (gamma .42), and having impregnated several women (gamma .61). All are plausible consequences of early exposure and habituation to frequent sex or of sociocultural or personality factors.

The current number of visiting mates, on the other hand, is related both to the man's (gamma .32) and his partner's educational level and to his being younger (gamma .30), but not to occupation or urban birth. It is not associated with the high fertility and male-dominance values with which cohabiting men tend to agree. This visiting group has frequent sexual intercourse (gamma .44) but tends to use effective contraception (gamma .38) and to be more positive about abortion (gamma .42). These are the least likely to have impregnated more than one woman (gamma − .36). The somewhat younger, more educated, literate, and higher-occupational-status males among the family planning clients, then—in contrast with those who are older, of lower socioeconomic status, and cohabiting—appear to be quite sexually active with more and better educated current visiting female partners whom they do not know very well, and with whom they try not to have babies. In this respect they (and their female partners) seem to be moving toward the sexual activity pattern of younger middle-class people in the industrialized world.

9 The Person in the Context

Affect, Competence, and Autonomy

Pamela L. at 23 can write something that is recognizable as her name. The world of printed words, however, conveys no information to her. "Me never learn," she said when I handed her a copy of the *Gleaner* after we had been together for an hour and a half. We had met at eight in the morning at the Manley Clinic, where she had brought her fourth child for "the belly-runnin" (diarrhea). She was fifth in line to see the doctor, the first woman identified by the nurse as sexually active without ever having used a contraceptive. When I approached, she looked down at the concrete floor. My first thought was that conversation might be difficult, especially if she felt I was too insistent. She brightened and agreed to talk with me, however, when I said I could arrange for her baby to be seen first.

Pamela was born and reared in rural St. Thomas. It was not expected that she should go to school past the third or fourth year: "Too much to be done at home." Her mother had died when she was very young, and she moved to Kingston at age 17 to find work and escape from a restrictive father and grandmother. At first she was a live-in domestic. Later, because her mistress "not treat me right," she found part-time employment doing housework by the day and moved into a tenement room. Although she had desired freedom she was lonely, fearful of attack, and now could not depend on food from her employer's kitchen. A man who lived nearby "came looking for me" one day. "Him said he care me," and soon they shared her room intermittently. Timid and withdrawn in the interview, she had the general manner of someone who felt herself small and defenseless in the face of an incomprehensible, hostile world. She dealt with this world by constricting and inhibiting herself, avoiding conflict, and being as inconspicuous as possible. Her part-time relationship with the man and the babies she had had for him gave her some security and a sense of engagement with others. A glimmer of self-aware-ness emerged as we talked together. She reluctantly acknowl-edged some resentful feelings toward her father for keeping her out of school to work, and toward her paternal grandmother for not having told her "about life," that is, about sex, reproduction, and contraception. Despite my expressions of interest, she remained silent about her man. I felt that she really did not want to confront herself as a person who, with effort, might be able to move out of the stream of seemingly inevitable events that would determine her life history. The man, who retained his own room (which she did not visit), provided her only consistent adult rela-tionship. It was, apparently, better not to examine this relation-ship too closely.

At first when I asked her to draw she said that she could not do so. But then she produced a tiny figure, barely recognizable as human, with no facial features except eyes. It had sticks for legs, no feet, and floated in a constricted segment of the upper left-hand corner of the paper. Upon questioning she hesitantly identi-fied it: "Her 'oman . . . not sure . . . maybe baby." Her response to a Thematic Apperception Test picture of an older woman and a young girl with a doll or baby was focused on the girl: "She not know what to do with her baby." At this point I asked if she, Pamela, had ever considered contraception. She had heard about "the planning" and knew that it was easily available; how-ever, she said, "Maybe later. Not ready yet." We then talked about what she might like to become, given the opportunity. Her aspirations were limited to finishing primary school and learning to be a seamstress—work she could do in her own home. She seemed defeated, with limited innate resources. Yet she did not reveal feelings of frustration so much as acceptance of life as it was, with herself a not totally comprehending or joyful, but none-theless participating part of it.

Pamela exemplified for me the Kingston slum woman whose life seems to drift, but in a manner shared by so many others as to constitute a collective pattern, part of the social structure.

She and others like her are excluded from the cultural main-stream of the educated upper and middle classes. Their behavior seems immediately determined by the need to act upon unpredict-able, concrete opportunities to enhance survival or take care of short-term needs. Her main connection with the long-term future is her children. Having children meets traditional expectations for early childbearing and large families. The modern emphasis on individual, sometimes lonely, responsibility for oneself and one's future is foreign to her. In these circumstances it is difficult to define the kind of behavior that might be regarded as self-determining or autonomous. For her, the meaning of such ideas as rational decision making, risk taking or planning for the future is unclear. The question arises: does Pamela's apparent passivity and willingness repeatedly to conceive children for whom she will be progressively less able to care reflect a basic incompe-tence? Given her illiteracy, is she innately limited? Or is this pat-tern of behavior and failure to learn primarily a consequence of the environment with which she has had to deal since childhood?

These are questions that might be raised about any of the non-literate women with whom we talked, or about those who after many partners are now burdened with children whom they must "pass on" to others to rear. It would be easy to conclude that they are relatively uniform, passive, dull, and socially incompe-tent. But more intimate contact belies this impression.

Self-Presentation

The nonliterates and the poorest women with the largest fami-lies interviewed for the study were as individually different as those who could read or write or who had somewhat more ade-quate support for their babies. It is not possible to distinguish most of the respondents on the basis of how they initially pre-sented themselves in the clinic. They varied in appearance and manner: their clothing ranged from plain, conservative, and dull to bright and lacy; shoes included flat rubber soles, conservative slippers, and high-heeled straps; hair was plaited or short, kinky, and close to the head; only a few had a well-developed "bush." Most wore few or no cosmetics, but some were gaudy with lipstick and blue or white eyeshadow. A few had costume jewelry.

In general, women who had dressed with more concern for the observer seemed more socially adept and comfortable. But some who had come plainly dressed were direct, poised, and cheerful. Others, more elaborately garbed, were anxious or flat and seemingly withdrawn.

The interview revealed other affective differences. Reactions to recalled sexual-reproductive events might be cheerful, depressed, or at least involved, or flat, neutral, and detached. Some produced early memories with alacrity; others were unable or unwilling to offer such memories to the interviewer. Some, in response to questions, readily categorized particular memories as "worst" or "best"; others said they were unable to do this. In every instance we probed as much as we dared, not wanting to risk alienation. Perhaps the fact that no respondent became sufficiently uncomfortable to leave or retreat into muteness indicates that we were too restrained.

Literacy

Approximately one-fifth of the women were not literate; they could do no more than read or write their name and make change. Education, as expected, accounts for most of the variance in this respect (gamma −.88). Their human figure drawings were primitive and fragmented (gamma .44). They tended to have been born in the country (gamma .40), reflecting the relative lack of schools and pressure to do agricultural work in childhood. The nonliterates as a group embraced the traditional matricentric attitudes most commonly encountered in rural women.

Being nonliterate is also associated with a reproductive life resembling that of people not educated past the primary level. Nonliterates tend not to delay their first or space later births (gamma

.38) and to have more pregnancies than others of similar age (gamma .39).

Mood and the Person

The typical respondent presented herself as reasonably cheerful, interested in the interviewer's questions, and quite willing to talk about herself. Just under one-fourth were identified by the interviewing psychiatrist as anxious. Only a few (11 percent) seemed overtly depressed. As the details of biography developed, however, general depressive preoccupations tended to emerge. The retrospective views of "flogging" and general childhood deprivation merged with the remembered shock of unexpected menarche. During the course of a reproductive career men were perceived increasingly as untrustworthy. Most conjugal unions without the support of legal marriage did not seem to be sources of emotional support or optimism. Although accumulating children were appreciated as sources of companionship and potential help in old age, increasing family size was associated with a wish that one did not have so many. The economic, emotional, social, and physical burdens of child rearing under precarious circumstances were never far from consciousness. Overall was a constant awareness of the fragility of one's socioeconomic and personal support system: jobs are scarce and low-paying; food, shelter, and clothing are expensive; gifts and small amounts of money from former mates who have fathered children, or even from the current conjugal partner, are irregular. The sole reference point for many, often involved in their journeying from city to country and back, was the extended group of female relatives with their children and their fluctuating male companions.

Approximately one-fifth of the women were described by the psychiatric interviewers as affectively flat. They tended to be less educated (gamma .37), unable to draw an integrated human figure (gamma .31), and believed in the grandmother's central role (gamma .65) and a preordained "lot" of children (gamma .39). They were not, however, older, country bred, or nonliterate. The highest correlation, that with a belief in the central role of the grandmother, is not indicative of rural, presumably more traditional, origins, belonging to the older (presumably less modern) generation, or nonliteracy. It is instead an indicator of having been "passed on" or of having been reared by a grandmother in lieu of a mother (see chapter 6). It is therefore not surprising that their histories revealed significant emotional and interpersonal features. Their communication with their first partner was poor (gamma .39), first coitus tended to be early (gamma .32), and they did not discuss contraception with their current mate (gamma .40). Perhaps a tendency to protect themselves by affective withdrawal allowed a relatively early, passive, and nonparticipant initiation into a sexual career. On the other hand, their tendency, despite an apparently traditional attitude toward their grandmother, to disagree significantly with the culturally prevalent positive attitudes to child care (gamma .43) and motherhood (gamma .41) suggests dissatisfaction with their lives and with their sexual-reproductive roles. It is plausible that this dissatisfaction, a probable consequence of sexual-reproductive experience, is rooted in the ambivalence of childhood. The ambivalence is revealed in the simultaneous centrality of positive attitudes to a grandmother's role and resentment at having been "given out" or "passed on" in early childhood to be reared by a grandmother or others. Respondents expressed this resentment in terms of diminished self-esteem, "embarrassment," "anger," or "being kept like slaves."

Women who reported no emotional intimacy with their first sexual partners and who did not communicate about sexual or contraceptive matters with their current mates tended to be anxious as well as affectively flat: they showed neither a cheerful nor a depressive response to life. They also tended to be suspiciously wary and distrustful of people with potential power. As one said, speaking of her dissatisfaction with various employers, "Them want to bring their voice over on top of you." Or another, speaking of her experience with men: "They don't come and explain that another girl friend has a baby for them, just tell lies." The short duration of the majority of their first unions permitted more (although not significantly so) subsequent unions and pregnancies.

Two women in the "flat" category left their mates after their babies had died, feeling there was nothing more to hold them together. Another would have liked to terminate her visiting union, which had persisted for three years with two pregnancies. She felt that the relationship was "drifting," but the man "won't leave me alone." Many of the "flat" women felt they had "no future" with their current mates, saying they did not even know their age, schooling, or occupation. Emotional unresponsiveness, lack of ordinary pleasure or sadness in conversation, may be one way in which these poor, powerless, and deprived people hide feelings of pessimism, worthlessness, inferiority, or depression from themselves.

Affective neutrality or the denial of feelings associated with memories of menarche or of first coitus characterized 24 percent and 14.7 percent of the 150 women, respectively. Affectively neutral or flat memories of first coitus in particular, as noted in chapter 6, are associated with a matricentric life view and not being satisfied with and not communicating with the current mate.

Affective flatness and the denial of early memories may be the responses of withdrawn, inadequate women to the interview itself. They can also be understood as a chronic way of dealing with stress. The denial of early memories in particular suggests that unresolved conflicts are dealt with at the cost of some personality constriction. Both affective withdrawal from the aspects of one's own interior life embodied in early memories and withdrawal from others, manifested in affective flatness, can reflect the operation of defensive processes. These defenses reduce the likelihood of affective arousal with its threat of disintegration or lack of control. This kind of repression, entailing the separation of affect from thoughts, is facilitated by the kind of life the respondents lived. Requiring attention to abrasive, concrete realities, it provides little enrichment and inhibits the development of creative fantasy. The fantasy that does emerge involves mainly the prospect of immediate gratification and protection through supplication, utilizing already available cultural vehicles in the form of belief in magic, witchcraft, and spirit-possession.

Aspirations

Whereas few respondents were satisfied with their current occupational status, most were relatively modest and traditional in terms of what they allowed themselves to prefer. Higher occupational aspirations were not associated with education nor with particular patterns of sexual or reproductive behavior. They varied independently and specifically with being reared by one's mother. Thus, the women who were most ambitious for themselves (and optimistic and self-confident) were not necessarily those who had already had the greatest school success. They might have had rather little schooling—although they did know how to read and write. Their most significant life experience was that of not having been "passed on" and thus of having been able to relate consistently until puberty with a natural mother for whom they were the object of primary affective interest.

Approximately one-fifth of the women might have aspired to a university education and almost three-fourths thought in terms of becoming a secretary, clerk, nurse, teacher, or some similar, traditionally female, white-collar worker. Relatively few, however, would actually have been interested in going back to school at this point. They were more ambitious for their daughters, with almost half looking to the university and almost all preferring one of the traditional female professions rather than a white-collar or clerical job. Almost one-third, though, believed that the daughter should make her own decisions about education and occupation. Aspirations for sons were somewhat higher than for daughters in terms of job status, but the difference was not impressive.

Thematic Apperception Test Cards

Xerox copies of five cards from the standard TAT test were presented to the respondents. The intent was to elicit organized associations to the pictures as indications of perceptual acuity and defense as well as attitudes toward life and people. The faces of the pictured characters had been blurred so that they were not obviously white; no respondent suggested that these portrayed white rather than black people. They were asked to tell a story about the picture on each, but were not urged to elaborate. The results, as with Rio de Janeiro *favelados* or Baltimore slumdwellers, tended to be sparse.

The first card is a picture of a person sitting on the floor, by a couch or bed. Responses were generally limited to a flat statement: "He sleeping" or "She crying" or "Man asleep" or "Woman crying." One-third of the 15 percent of the figures designated as male were described as asleep or resting. Almost two-thirds of the 60 percent designated female were described as crying. In one-fourth of the cases no reference was made to gender identity, and in 40 percent there was no reference to emotions.

The next picture shows two people at the foot of some stairs. They are sometimes referred to as "a couple," fighting or talking; occasionally as a mother and daughter; most frequently as two women angry with each other or fighting. The large majority of respondents (79 percent), however, made no reference to emotions.

The third card, showing a woman embracing a man and looking up at him while he looks away, was invariably seen as a male and female couple, most often in some kind of adversary relationship, such as "He not hearing her," but occasionally in a positive or lovemaking situation. Here, too, although there were references to the acts of pleading-rejecting (33 percent), lovemaking (19 percent), comforting, or quarreling (14 percent), there was no explicit reference to the feeling or emotion of the actors in 75 percent of the responses.

The fourth card, a scene with an older and younger female, the latter holding an infant or doll, was always identified as describing a girl and a woman, sometimes merely as an adult and child. These were most often described as a mother and daughter (24 percent), occasionally as a grandmother and daughter. The small figure was seen variously as a doll or a baby or was completely ignored. Although there were references to the older woman counseling (25 percent) or pleading (19 percent) and to the "daughter" rejecting her advice (11 percent), there was no specific reference to the actors' feelings or emotions in 76 percent of the responses.

The last card shows three people. A young woman holding books and apparently dressed for school or town is in the foreground. To one side an apparently pregnant woman in a flowing gown leans against a tree. At the center is a shirtless man, his back to the viewer, with a horse. Beyond are farm buildings and fields. Some respondents saw the people only as individuals, some as a family. The largest number (39 percent) identified the young woman with books as a "daughter" going to school. Forty percent made no reference to any specific person or act, and 73 percent did not refer to feeling or emotion. Most (81 percent) made no reference to the apparent pregnancy. This is a pattern of denial or scotomization of people or their affective significance —in this instance of pregnancy-related figures.

In general the women tended to ignore many of the characters and to circumscribe their view of the pictures, referring only to a single person or a couple. Even for these there was little mention of personal roles or actions. The figures were described as sad, unhappy, crying, or angry, but the great majority of respondents make no reference to feelings or emotions. The unique evocativeness of the first picture may be related to the isolation of its central figure. Several respondents commented "She all alone" or "Not know what to do now" or "Feeling bad and no one to help her."

There are no consistently significant correlations between TAT responses and socioeconomic status. Women reporting that they had no meaningful communication with the man with whom they first had intercourse tended to see the TAT figures as depressed and passive (gammas .19, .31, .43). The relative few who did have satisfactory communication with their first partner tended to see cheerful, optimistic, or active behavior (gammas .33, .24, .24, .24). Those who wished that they had fewer children (were dissatisfied with their current procreative status) also tended to see figures who were sad, crying, or unhappy (gamma .29).

These correlations may suggest the persisting effect of an earlier unsatisfying experience and its sequelae. Or, as in the case of affective flatness, personal problems and attitudes might determine the quality both of the first experience and of the later TAT interpretation. It is plausible that a girl who is passive, apathetic, or depressed could allow herself to be "forced" or at least persuaded with minimal affective involvement into having intercourse under less than optimal emotional circumstances. It is also possible, however, that an initial unhappy experience might lead one to expect if not to experience the worst, and thus increase the likelihood that fantasies produced in response to the TAT pictures (and real-life stimuli) would involve a projection of herself; that is, she would tend to see unhappy people upon whom life imposes experiences that they cannot or do not try to manage.

Draw-a-Person Performance

At the end of the interview each woman was asked to draw a human figure, and then another of the opposite sex. Afterward she was asked to comment on her drawings: Who were they? Of whom did they remind her? What were they doing, thinking, and feeling?

Thirty-two of the respondents refused to draw, including several at the Manley Clinic who said they did not wish to put down the babies in their arms. The majority of the pictures thus came from women with sufficient initiative and self-concern to be JFPA clients. Sixty percent of those who did cooperate first drew female figures. No consistent differences between the first and second figure appeared when a preliminary sample was scored, and the following descriptions are therefore confined to the first drawing.

Responses to the inquiry about the drawings were sparse. Only 79 of the 118 women who drew noted the affective state of the figure. Of these, 62 percent referred in some way to the unhappiness, sickness, or pessimism of the person drawn. Poor school marks, illness, and lack of work, money, or success were recurrent themes. Love or companionship were mentioned rarely. The word "unhappy" appeared at times to include a feeling of anger. The other 38 percent referred to the person as smiling, cheerful, or happy.

Some sample unhappy responses:

"A nine-year-old boy . . . doing nothing . . . The street windy . . . He not happy . . . poor school marks."

"A 20-year-old man . . . Reminds me my husband . . . bad . . . sick . . . not happy."

"A woman . . . me . . . upset because no money . . . Her wanting for money."

"A 25-year-old man . . . standing . . . doing nothing . . . maybe thinking how he get a little work . . . sad . . . He needs food."

"A 30-year-old woman . . . standing . . . sad and gloomy . . . has the flu . . . Maybe her man not want her because she not working."

"A 25-year-old man . . . a gardener . . . thinking about money . . . not too happy . . . Maybe his woman don't want him because he a gardener."

"A 10-year-old girl . . .me . . . standing there . . . unhappy, not well, thinking too hard, life will be hard, no success."

"A 30-year-old woman . . . me, crying, sad, too many children, not well . . . The future has nothing for her."

"A 40-year-old woman . . . thinking about the changes in life . . . experiencing worse things now than she used to."

Some of those considered currently unhappy may have had a better future outlook:

"A 30-year-old woman . . . unhappy . . . but her future is good . . . She stands with pride."

"A 25-year-old woman . . . sad, doing nothing . . . hopes future will be brighter . . . She concentrating."

Some sample happy responses:

"A 25-year-old man . . . my boy friend . . . He thinking about me, love."

"A 20-year-old woman . . . She smiling . . . don't know why."

"A nine-year-old boy . . . like my son . . . playful, happy."

"A 20-year-old man, my cousin, laughing, happy, wants to be comfortable financially, trying to save."

"An 80-year-old woman . . . happy . . . She prepare her soul to go to heaven."

"A 35-year-old man . . . He go around giving people children . . . He happy . . . He will take a woman who will look after him and marry her . . . but they keep many things to themselves."

Some sample responses not including a clear affective statement:

"A 34-year-old woman . . . self . . . sitting in office . . . thinking about getting advice."
"A five-year-old boy . . . standing."

Almost half the drawings were either so primitive as to be hardly recognizable as human or were stick figures with stereotyped and partial faces. Most prominent were missing or distorted limbs (61.9 percent) and missing or distorted secondary sex characteristics (61 percent). More than half lacked or had only vestigial or distorted sense organs, and almost half were tiny, occupying a very small part of the page, or huge, with boundaries at the edges of the page. Twenty-three percent were not clearly human. Only 7.5 percent were well proportioned, detailed, and unequivocally drawn.

These were scored according to a system based on Harris (1963). Low-scoring drawings tend to be those with many distortions and omissions, especially in relation to a clear gender identification, often not clearly human. Absence or distortion in one area tends to be associated with similar deficits in others. More than two-thirds scored at a level of three or less, regarded in the United States as associated with psychotic and mentally retarded children (Harris, 1963).

The higher-scoring, better integrated, more mature drawings were produced by the literate (gamma .44), better educated (gamma .54) women who had engaged in early purposeful contraception (gamma .39). The lower-scoring, poorly integrated, primitive drawings belonged to those who were older (gamma .30); had more visiting mates per age group (gamma .35) and more impregnators per pregnancy (gamma .30); believed, traditionally, in a preordained "lot" of children (gamma .44); and had more often passed on children to be reared by others (gamma .44). Inability to produce an adequate drawing is also associated with affective flatness during the interview (gamma .34) and the denial of earliest memories (gamma .47). These women were not, however, of rural birth or low economic level as revealed by poor housing. The question remains whether their inability to project themselves in an adequate drawing is a reflection of little education, of a more basic lack of affective or cognitive competence, or of defense systems utilizing denial and repression and inhibiting perceptual accuracy and creativity. A failure of emotional integration could interfere with the ability to portray an intact human being of appropriate size with limbs, sense organs, and secondary sex characteristics placed in a field of potential action. The fragmented, floating figures, swollen or microscopic, haphazardly placed on the paper, restricted to a corner or poorly contained by the page, and of indeterminate or incomplete gender, may all reflect emotional constriction and affective flatness resulting from lack of the social and cognitive expansion provided by education. These bodies are lived in a context of conflict and discouragement.

Autonomy, Defense, and Coping

The women who are JFPA clients have decided, however late in life, to manage their own fertility by technical methods. It is clear that the decision may not be permanent and that the attempt may be transient. They may nonetheless be considered less willing to submit to the pressures of biology and society, and more autonomous and independent than their peers who never make the effort and let nature take its course. But the assumption of autonomous tendencies need not imply capacity to cope. Using technical contraceptive methods is not culturally perceived as "natural," and behaving in an "unnatural" way may not represent healthy self-management for people who are comfortable in a system of beliefs and values in which procreation and fertility have a central place. Thus, early contraceptors could be regarded as culturally deviant or marginal rather than as adequately coping people.

Culturally supported socioeconomic considerations could also discourage a view of noncontraception as a failure in coping, autonomy, or competence. For working-class women growing up within a "culture of motherhood," a sense of self-determination and strength could be expressed in traditional ways: producing a maximum number of children and, with them, creating one's own enclave and source of security. This is adaptive behavior in a potentially hostile environment in which no one but children and mothers can be trusted. If it assumes the capacity to feed and otherwise care adequately for the children, such behavior can also bespeak optimism and self-esteem. The opposing view is that of the industrialized, educated segment of the world: the production of many children in insecure economic circumstances reflects a present rather than a future orientation, lack of capacity to appreciate reality, or simply denial or failure to realize that one's children may have defective chances for optimal development. In one sense this may be regarded as a failure in empathy: if a woman perceives her children primarily as a source of her own ultimate security, she exhibits a utilitarian rather than an empathic attitude toward them and toward the men whom she allows to impregnate her.

This position can be supported by human figure drawings, a mosaic design test, and the Rorschach, administered to a group of Jamaican children aged 7 to 16 in the late 1940s (Kerr, 1952). These children were said to "live in an environment which does not allow them either free or controlled expression of their personalities." They "become more introversive [with age] . . . Energy which could be used creatively becomes inhibited . . . [They] lack initiative and often become apathetic after the age of 11 or 12" (p. 189). In addition, Rorschach results suggested that the children had "not developed their potential capacity for logical thought to its full extent" (p. 190). These characteristics were attributed to confused patterns of early family relations, economic frustration, color prejudice, limited educational opportunities, and to the availability and social encouragement of magical beliefs.

Similar characteristics of our adult sample, spanning a range of educational and occupational achievement, with two-thirds actively engaged in an effort to regulate their own fertility, are suggested by the generally impoverished TAT stories, in which affect tends to be ignored, and by the generally primitive and poorly integrated human figure drawings. Moreover, the group subdivides naturally as characteristics cluster together. Thus, the women least capable of producing an integrated human figure drawing tended to be those who showed affective flatness, denied the existence of earliest memories, were nonliterate, and more often subscribed to such traditional folk beliefs as a fore-ordained "lot" of children. These are features often associated with a deficit in the capacity for creative imagination, in contrast with the active use of existing folk myths as a ready-made basis for behavior. This deficit bears on the capacity for self-regulation, which invariably involves projecting oneself into the future and into other social contexts. Limited capacity to draw an integrated figure appears to be the key feature in this cluster; it expresses the deficits in self-conception and creative imagination with which the other features are correlated. It is also the only one positively correlated at a high level of significance with high partner diversity, high reproductive performance, and a high incidence of passing one's children on to others to be reared. If, as seems probable, competence in drawing figures and ability to read and write reflect some mixture of innate capacity and developmental experience, they may be antecedent to early coitus, many partners, and many children. In this sense, these qualities contribute to a woman's being "at risk" for producing many children under unfavorable support circumstances.

Given the assumption that effective fertility regulation reflects an attempt to achieve personal autonomy, willingness to use technical methods may be viewed as part of a general pattern of belief and action. This pattern includes the tendency to act decisively and to accomplish clearly defined, nontraditional goals (which may be culturally alien yet perceived as personally useful) with the most effective available means. It requires differentiating oneself from others to the extent that individual needs and aims are perceived as separate. A sense of personal boundaries and self-worth, apart from the worth of the community of which one is a part, are essential to this kind of individuation and differentiation. It requires, as well, freedom from fear of isolation, rejection, or extrusion from the group.

In some respects these characteristics are found in persons defined as modern in contrast to traditional. They cope rather than adjust. They are open both to new ways of perceiving and construing the world and to new methods and techniques for achieving goals. They are not bound by old views and approaches and are not made anxious by the prospect of abandoning them. They do not require children for their psychosocial security or as means of self-affirmation or of demonstrating environmental control through the processes of impregnation and delivery. Such attitudes of activity rather than passivity, of achieving through personal effort rather than supplication, are part of the modern value system. They also imply a willingness to trust others (as well as oneself) and the capacity to experience failure or frustration without assigning the blame to outside forces. In addition, they suggest a capacity to feel connected with common aims through abstract and symbolic rather than concrete means.

These modern characteristics, however, have not formerly had survival value in the tight, family-oriented, peasant communities of the small island. Traditional values have helped integrate people who, without money or technology, have had to depend on one another for food, shelter, and communal security, including a sense of worth. Children were among the means of perpetuating the community and its values. Reliance upon the group and not acting apart from it were essential to acceptance by others and to the maintenance of a personal support system.

Symptomatic Sex and Reproduction

Regulating one's own fertility, an instance of self-management, requires adequate personality resources as well as available services. It implies the capacity to perceive oneself as distinct from the sociocultural context and its constraints, and the self-confidence to imagine a more satisfying future separate from this context.

Many women coming for contraception, even after several

pregnancies, intimated this capacity in their earlier relations with men. A higgler in her late twenties, for example, had sexual intercourse for the first time at age 18 because she "loved him and wanted it." But after legal marriage to her first partner, followed by the birth of five children, she left him. She said she "had expected to work with him to better ourselves," but was disappointed by his lack of ambition. She had stayed with him because she thought it wrong to break up a legal marriage. She finally made up her mind to separate when she discovered that he had a visiting woman by whom he had two children. Eventually she hopes to emigrate: "In Jamaica women really have it hard. Men give nothing for the pickney, woman must go away to advance herself."

Despite little schooling this woman was able to draw two well-organized human figures. The female figure "feels the man is not behaving, she doesn't tell him that she is going to family planning. The man feels she should feel good toward him. Separately, they work. Together, they do sex."

Sexual intercourse, like any other behavior, may be considered symptomatic under certain circumstances. Symptomatic acts reflect or stand for an underlying process that is out of awareness, and thus out of conscious control. The process may involve a tension-generating conflict resulting in efforts at defense; such a defense might take the form of keeping a wish or impulse out of consciousness in order to reduce one's anxiety or guilt to a manageable level. To the degree that motives or aims are unconscious, they do not fit the person's explicit goals or philosophy of life. Symptomatic behaviors are maladaptive. They do not help to establish and maintain a stable, reciprocal, and need-satisfying relationship between a person and his environment. They are usually, though not always—and sometimes after the fact—experienced as distressing, painful, or alien by the actor. Their repetitive, obligatory quality stems precisely from these features: if a person acts in search of unconscious goals or is driven mainly by unconscious motives, the search is bound to be continued and repeated. It recurs in one context after another and with one person after another because its object is not defined. It can never be achieved. The process itself may then acquire the characteristics of a goal, and the result, however unwanted, is discounted so long as the person is involved in the process. A cognitive structure of thoughts and expectations, historically and symbolically determined, develops with repetition and gives the process meaning. This is a meaning beyond its original symbolic, conflict-resolving, tension-reducing, or compromising functions that permit the disguised gratification, for example, of some unacceptable wish or aim. The behavior tends increasingly to occur in contexts and in response to circumstances different from those that originally activated it. It can itself become the consummatory act, relieving tension and providing a sense of temporary fulfillment (regardless of the secondary distress and subjective sense of it as alien) following a variety of needful private experiences. Sexual intercourse, for example, may be sought when feelings of loneliness, powerlessness, rootlessness, or inexpressible and not fully conscious anger at an important other demand relief and cannot be dealt with by direct action. The private state in these instances may be experienced as sexual need, frustration, or deprivation; but the personal interpretation of the impulse to action as sexual may have begun originally as an attempt to resolve quite different conflicts or to deal with different needs. It comes from the new anticipatory meanings that the act has acquired over time and through repetition. Similarly, having a baby (or the idea of having a baby) might have had such original symptomatic meanings as taking revenge against a mother, displacing her as the central reproductively mature female in the household, using a man instrumentally, or demonstrating that one could produce a child without a man's involvement. But despite these origins, the baby-producing acts or their anticipation may develop a new structure of meaning. Sexual intercourse without contraception, with the implication that pregnancy is possible although not inevitable, may itself become a consummatory act to be regretted only when pregnancy or the new baby begins to constrain personal freedom and add to already difficult social and economic burdens.

One version of this kind of life history is that of a woman with more security than most. Now 33, she has had four children by the same man, with whom, after 11 years of cohabitation, she is expecting marriage. Her first coitus at age 18 was a painful, frightening rape by an older boarder in a house where she worked as a domestic. She spoke of it to no one because she was afraid of losing her job. At 21, however, two years after having moved to Kingston, she met a man several years her senior, an odd-job carpenter with a primary school education. He was kind, made no demands, and gave her a sense of security. They had intercourse, her first experience since the rape—she reported it as mildly pleasant because "it make him happy"—and decided to live together. She became pregnant within three months. During pregnancy she was "not sad or happy." This resembled her feeling at unexpected menarche (about which mother told her nothing) at age 14: "I had no feeling, but knew that I wouldn't go to a man because I didn't want to have a baby at that young age." When she had her first child, she felt as she did after succeeding deliveries: "I might be sorry before, but after I make myself contented since it happen already." After the first baby, because neither she nor her mate had a job they agreed that they should postpone another. She did obtain a diaphragm from JFPA, but it was too late; they had been having intercourse several times a week (she still experienced no physical pleasure but felt "taken care of") and she was already pregnant. The next pregnancy was delayed by three years. Her mate went to Cuba to find work, but in his intervals at home every three or four months they had frequent intercourse without contraception. When she did become pregnant she was "fretful" but accepted the baby: "There nothing else to do." After that, by mutual consent, they tried coitus interruptus. But he found it a "strain" and she "felt sorry for him." A fourth pregnancy ensued. This time she was very unhappy and after delivery she decided to get a diaphragm. But "somehow," she said, "I just did not go." She finally came, at the time of the research interview, one month after the spontaneous abortion of her fifth pregnancy: "To be truthful I glad I lost it . . . Now I like to have something that I can control myself." She noted that she preferred sons to daughters because boys could not become pregnant.

This woman's drawings were huge and amorphous, filling the pages with faint wobbly lines with gaps between them. The first is a man "not doing anything . . . sad . . . makes me feel sad, like out of a job. Not well in his mind. He empty, needs food." The other figure was a 33-year-old woman, herself, thinking about getting advice: "Maybe they will sleep together." On the TAT card she identified herself with the girl: "She not happy with her baby."

This woman's repeated, seemingly unwanted, pregnancies despite her knowledge of contraception fit the cultural blueprint. Yet the data suggest a symptomatic quality to the action pattern. She dealt with the potentially overwhelming menarchal experience, being raped, and then her first pregnancy by excluding any feeling from consciousness. Each event was described in flat, neutral terms. She seemed to perceive herself as insubstantial, with poorly defined boundaries, "empty," and in danger of loss of control at the hands of outside forces. She dealt with this, hypothetically, by placating her mate—the symbol of these forces—giving him what he wanted, and in so doing filled her own emptiness and gave herself an identity, however reluctantly, as a loving and forgiving mate, a fertile woman, and a mother. The achievement of a sense of boundaries was essential to her gradually evolving concept of her body as something not just operated by nature or by others, but by herself.

Motivations for behavior that lie outside one's awareness impair personal autonomy to the extent that they tie individual acts, thoughts, and feelings to the biographical past and to the swarming wishes, fantasies, and imagery of the unconscious. They also subject the person to the bondage imposed by the consequences of repeated symptomatic acts, in this instance the accumulating children resulting from repeated uncontracepted coitus. The need to prove one's fertility and the wish for large families have historical and socioeconomic origins; reluctance to contracept, especially by men but often by women as well, continues to reflect some of these variables. But although they result in part from the environmental background and in part from personal familial experience, uncontracepted intercourse and pregnancy also have individual symptomatic aspects. When a pattern reflects both the sociocultural and the individual psychobiographical streams, it is especially hard to discover the latter. The occurrence of individual symptomatic acts is reinforced to the degree that they represent expected, socially sanctioned ways of behaving and hence become ego-syntonic. In a context of collective approval, self-awareness rarely develops until the cumulative consequences of the act produce sufficient psychological pain to force conscious recognition of one's pattern of behaving as essentially self-destructive.

10 Public Policy and Private Behavior

Banana With Too Many Suckers Can't Fat!
National Family Planning Board advertisement

Put It Back With Dragon Stout!
Newspaper advertisement

The Social Context of Reproductive Experience

Sexual intercourse, pregnancy, and having babies are activities common to people in all settings, regardless of social and cultural context. But the contexts in which these tendencies emerge into consciousness determine the nature of their expression and give them specific meaning. The context influences the ways in which the activities become part of apprehended and reflected upon individual experience.

Socioeconomic Organization and Cultural Integrity

The socioeconomic matrix of personal reproductive behavior in Jamaica, as in many developing societies, is still postcolonial, characterized by an uneven transition from a plantation to a business, manufacturing, and tourist economy. It is difficult in a transitional setting to achieve the significant sharing of important symbols and values that is necessary for cultural integrity and national identity. Continuing emigration in pursuit of personal goals or a better life, from country to town or overseas, has kept interpersonal and community ties weak. For many Jamaicans, moving away has been the only avenue for improvement; as a result, the possible abandonment of familiar relationships has been a regular expectation.

The major unifying forces in most plantation societies were religious belief and imposed colonial power. Religious belief required supplication as a means of achieving personal tranquility, although it permitted some energetic and charismatic individuals to achieve social power outside the context of daily working life. Imposed colonial power minimized opportunity for the oppressed classes to identify with their masters. The vestiges of an era of coerced labor and disenfranchisement of the majority may still interfere with the growth of cultural integrity (Mintz, 1966). Emancipation allowed at least some members to identify with the dominant social system. As in the United States, however, the colonial rulers constituted an emulative reference group to which workers could never hope fully to belong. The white masters owned the culture; the black workers acquired distorted fragments or accommodated to it. Adherence to the dominant standards, therefore, even for those who seemed most thoroughly acculturated, was never fully rewarded. It is probable that even the most Europeanized West Indians, conscious of discrimination, however subtle, felt ambivalence for their white models.

When each country attained independence, nationalism became a new integrating force. In the mid-1970s in particular a new political emphasis began to emerge in Jamaica. Without severing its symbolic ties to Britain the controlling political party began vigorously pursuing its ties to Third World nations in a deliberate move toward establishing a new national identity. Such a development could in time allow a state and economy to "impose themselves . . . upon traditional social situations." The state presents itself as "a mobilizing agent for development . . . a symbol of . . . collective aspirations" easier for people to identify with than the economic system, "a vehicle of their social ambitions instead of an inhibiting structure" (Berger, Berger, and Kellner, 1974, p. 127). One means of establishing an effective government fertility policy could be the transformation of a peasant people into a collectivity. A new national consciousness based on political rather than purely economic development might make personal aspirations (in this instance an ideal family size) identical with those of the state. This move, however, like most other deliberate efforts to attain social or cultural integrity by political means, was attempted in a context of marginality. Jamaican working-class men and women at the beginning of the 1980s still appear to have one foot in each of two cultures and suffer from uncertainty of belonging (Stonequist, 1973; Park, 1950). The two cultures, though complicated by color distinctions, are those found in most developing countries: the rural, traditional, past-oriented, nontechnological, religious-supplicant culture of poverty depending upon oral history and socially inherited ways of doing things; and the urban, modern, future-oriented, technological, secular culture of the more economically secure, depending upon written history, communications, and making decisions at a variety of choice points instead of upon social inheritance. The division also remains between the culture of women and the culture of men. This is significantly expressed in attitudes toward sex, conjugal partnerships, and producing and being responsible for children.

Distrust and an everyone-for-himself view are found in deprived communities throughout the world. The lack of communication, however, and the economic wariness of members of a conjugal couple or sexual partnership in relation to each other have been especially striking in Jamaica. Our female respondents suggested that many couples fear competition from each other, even for food, work, or privileges. This lack of mutual trust apparently has not changed significantly in more than a generation. Cohen (1955) reported that most couples felt themselves unhappily married, having entered into the union for economic security that did not materialize. Mates did not share their leisure, and if sexual relations were unsatisfactory either could seek a new partner—without dissolving the household—with only little expectation of community censure. This style of conjugal life fits the lack of a developed community spirit described by Wagley (1957) as part of "plantation America." He reported a general lack of community cohesion and organization similar to what Mintz

(1966) viewed as an aspect of the "individualization" of Caribbean peoples. Mintz saw this reflected in the fragility of sexual unions as well as the generally shallow nature of kinship systems that recognize few relationships and rarely act in concert on issues of common interest. He regards as a major basis of social interaction among the rural lower-class Caribbean peoples their ability to establish dyadic relationships aimed at satisfying particular individual needs. In this view radial sets of two-person linkages are more significant for social action than are groups formed around institutions and interacting in terms of kinship rights and obligations. The history of this relational pattern includes the worker's need on traditional plantations to pantomime dependency as a means of gaining essential favors from the owner (Wolf, 1959).

Modernization and Reproductive Behavior:
Promise and Paradox

A national policy requiring voluntary limitation of personal options does not thrive in an environment in which people cannot identify with common symbols, ideals, and goals. Effective implementation requires converting an aggregate of individuals into a social system, developing reciprocal feelings of trust and responsibility, and fostering a commitment to action on the basis of a shared value system. One route to social organization and cultural integrity is modernization.

Structural, institutional modernization is associated with mass education, urbanization, industrialization, and extension of the mass media (Miller and Inkeles, 1974). These provide bases for new types of individual learning and work experience, producing in turn new ways of thinking, feeling, and acting.

Employment in particular is essential to the self-esteem and feeling of belonging necessary for identification with national purpose and policy. Socialization into the status of salaried or regularly employed worker can engender identification as a member of a group with a sense of power to be achieved from collective effort (Brody, 1973). The expectation of regular wages from an impersonal source, acceptance of the new worker's status, and the knowledge and sense of mastery stemming from education and literacy have, in many industrializing countries, contributed to a transformation in the styles of thinking, perceiving, and evaluating the world: "As modernization proceeds, there is a transformation both in the organization of knowledge and in cognitive style, in what is known and in how it is known" (Berger, Berger, and Kellner, 1974).

Inkeles's (1969) psychological modernity syndrome includes such items as subjective efficacy, openness to change, high value placed on planning and punctuality, valuing equal rights for women, autonomy in the face of kinship obligations, and accepting the findings of modern science. Education is most important in producing this syndrome; urban residence has almost no independent effect (Inkeles and Smith, 1974).

Attitudes and feelings favoring self-determination, activity rather than passivity in the face of external influence, and recourse to technology rather than religion can all be considered reflections of individual psychological modernity. This "modern" self-concept is natural for the person whose ordinary, everyday life reinforces his or her awareness of a capacity for self-determination and independence from the inhibiting influence of poverty. It follows the ancient Greek image of civilized man who, like the gods, makes his own destiny. It contrasts sharply with the lack of information and exclusion from the symbolic-meaningful experience of the dominant culture (Brody, 1966, 1968) that characterize slumdwellers throughout the world.

Data from East Pakistan, India, Israel, and Nigeria suggest that structural change in institutions has little effect on the acceptance of birth limitation "without intervening psychic change in individuals" (Miller and Inkeles, 1974, p. 183). Higher living standards, in contrast to education and occupation, seem to have no independent effect upon modernity. The most powerful stimulus to developing modern attitudes is extensive contact with modern institutions leading to belief in the value of science, technology, and medicine. Inherent in such beliefs, we assume, is the confidence of individuals that they can acquire control over their environments and manage their own destinies. The possibly illusory nature of such confidence remains an uninvestigated factor in determining patterns of illness or discomfort in modern men.

Confidence in one's capacity for environmental mastery or management of one's own destiny should be revealed in actions as well as in attitudes. Significant discrepancies have been reported in Jamaica between expressed desires to contracept and to limit family size and the actual use of contraceptives when they were provided (K. A. Smith, 1971). More research has been done elsewhere. In Bangladesh, for example, from 1965 to 1974, the large proportion of people who had acquired family planning knowledge and the widely expressed wish to limit family size contrasted sharply with the actual level of contraceptive use (Huber and Khan, 1979). In 1968-1969, although 55 percent of rural and 62 percent of urban women said they wanted no more children, only 1.9 and 3.7 percent, respectively, were actually using modern methods (Pakistan Family Planning Council, 1973). In 1975 a house-to-house contraceptive distribution program to married couples in rural Bangladesh villages resulted in an estimated 11 to 17 percent drop in fertility over a four-month period, particularly in 25-to-39-year-old women who already had five or more children (Huber and Khan, 1979). Having noted earlier studies demonstrating the difficulty of maintaining momentum in a new program, the authors recommended a variety of available techniques, especially injectables and sterilization, promoted by intensive fieldwork with younger married women who had higher social status than the visiting workers previously used.

Individual differences in the capacity for self-determination have been related to conceptions of self as either a "pawn" or an "origin" of social causation (DeCharms, 1968) and to an expectation of the outcome of personal action as internally or externally controlled (Rotter, 1966). Evidence of high internal control characterized unmarried female undergraduates who contracepted, and a "sense of efficacy" (Williamson, 1969) has similarly been related to favorable attitudes toward regulating one's fertility. That these factors may, however, have roots independent of socioeconomic status is suggested in a report that lower-class black couples who used contraceptives were discriminated from a matched group of nonusers on the basis of tests of feelings of efficacy, need for achievement (in men), and a tendency to plan ahead (Keller, Sims, Henry, and Crawford, 1970). M. B. Smith, who has summarized and reinterpreted these and related studies (1972, 1973), perceives "a cluster of self-attitudes that tend to function as a self-fulfilling prophecy. People who are convinced that they are 'origins,' that their important outcomes are under their own control, behave so as to enhance the likelihood that their beliefs will be confirmed; so, unfortunately, do those who see themselves as 'pawns' at the mercy of external forces" (Smith, 1973, p. 14).

People who may be considered modern on the basis of socio-economic status, urban residence, occupation, and education are also "more likely to value a conjugal relationship that is more flexible, verbal, and egalitarian" (Fawcett and Bornstein, 1973, p. 111). Communication between couples, valuing the woman's needs for personal mobility and growth, and the protection of her body from the effects of multiple pregnancy would logically seem to promote the planned use of contraception to delay, space, and eventually limit reproduction. Although becoming modern is not solely a matter of achieving adequate education and employment, these help people to acquire a personal sense of power, freedom, and thus the ability to trust new experience and ideas (Brody, 1974). The current ritual aspects of Jamaican student-teacher interaction are likely to be replaced by active learning and seeking. Traditional acceptance of natural givens will be replaced by the expectation that technologically informed effort can in fact modify the course of natural events. As a corollary, the family planning message—which currently offers the deceptive promise that fewer children will necessarily result in a better life—should achieve greater validity. Modernization should eventually lead to the extinction of the "culture of motherhood."

Our more educated respondents, both male and female, did adhere less to traditional beliefs and attitudes and were more favorable to women's autonomy and freedom to regulate their fertility. There is, however, much variation in respect to these issues among the less educated group of respondents. People classified according to various indexes of "modernity" vary in their attitudes, feelings, actions, and the quality of their life experience. Individual differences in innate capacities, competence, and the experience of early parental relationships as well as other aspects of personal biography seem more significant determinants among people without education. For those lower-socioeconomic-status and ethnically isolated groups with the highest fertility, these differences are significant.

The most recent reports (Dunnell, 1979; Digest, 1980) confirm the persistence of socioeconomic class differences in reproductive-contraceptive behavior for women in stable sexual partnerships within modern, industrialized societies. In the 1970s, for example, among women then aged 40 to 49, 55 percent of British women within the two lowest occupational groups, compared with 41 percent of those in the two highest, had engaged in unprotected premarital sexual intercourse. Among women aged 20 to 30, only 30 and 10 percent, respectively, had had unprotected premarital sex with their husbands. The data on premarital conception are comparable. Among women in the two highest socioeconomic classes in the 1966-1970 marriage cohort, only 8 percent were pregnant at the time of marriage, in contrast to 28 percent of those in the two lowest. In the 1971-1975 marriage cohort the incidence had dropped to 4 and 25 percent, respectively. These data underrepresent the actual proportion of premarital pregnancies in a context in which it is clear that abortion is underreported: a comparison of statistics indicated that with an average notified abortion rate of 132 per 1,000 live births, women in the sample reported only 62 per 1,000.

Of perhaps greater significance for Jamaica are data on unmarried British women. Of those conceiving between 1970 and 1974, 58 percent married in order to legitimize the birth and 28 percent terminated the pregnancy. In the United States, 37 percent of premarital pregnancies among teenagers and 50 percent among those aged 20-24 were terminated by abortion (O'Connell and Moore, 1980). These figures illustrate the differences between countries in value systems and in availability of legal abortion. Differences in willingness to abort, however, remain tied to social class. In England among women in nonmanual occupational classes (presumably more "modern" and self-determining) 45 percent of all nonmarital conceptions ended in abortion, miscarriage, or stillbirth, compared with only 19 percent of women in manual or unskilled classes.

A subjective sense of competence and autonomy, of separate identity and self-esteem seems important for the effective employment of technical devices to regulate bodily processes hitherto left to nature. Some working-class Jamaican women achieve this competence and confidence with progressive life experience, but often not before they have already burdened themselves with children to whom they cannot give optimal care. Accordingly, it seems unlikely that more exposure to schools and to scientific-technical values espoused in the media or by social and national leaders can achieve psychological modernization so long as a person belongs to a group that has no actual social power. Within such groups the abrasive conditions of life interfere with the optimal realization of latent abilities during early development, and these conditions remain in adulthood as a daily reminder of one's inferior, deprecated, and powerless status. Moreover, values are acquired and particular ways of behaving reinforced by significant others within the same (normative or comparative) reference group. Even within the confines of socioeconomic powerlessness, however, it may be possible to increase the likelihood of private mastery over one's own fertility and thus, in time, the achievement of greater individual freedom. Such a development would require more deliberate attention by planners to dealing with the psychocultural aspects of personal fertility control separately from the socioeconomic context. With this approach, autonomy and separateness would become less important than cultural and interpersonal solidarity expressed in learning processes, contraceptive usages, and relationships that accord with traditional perceptions of what is right, valued, proper, and natural.

It is clear that structural modernization of a country does not necessarily result in personal modernization for the most reproductively active individuals in the least stable conjugal relationships. Moreover, it may even have corollaries that are regressive in terms of individual management of health, reproduction, and personal relationships. Recent reports, for example, suggest that an increase in infant malnutrition is associated with earlier weaning and increased use of processed formulas or condensed milk in the Jamaican working-class community. Whereas in 1947 no mothers were reported to have weaned their infants before the age of five months, 25 percent were reported to have done so in 1971-1974, and breast feeding has declined among Kingston mothers (Landman et al., 1976). The effect of this decline upon fertility is uncertain, but it is probably inimical to the physical health of infants and to mother-infant bonding. These changes may be viewed in part as a response to commercial advertising associated with the development of Jamaica as a market for industrial products, in part as evidence of Jamaican women's increased acceptance of technology. They are also understandable as an adaptation to a social reality requiring young mothers to work away from home whenever limited opportunity presents itself. Work in factories, businesses without child care facilities, buses and the cabs of trucks, strange upper-class homes, and tasks requiring strenuous physical effort make continued regular lactation difficult.

Private Experience in the Public Context

Private biography as well as public context determines the nature of activity and the significance of current experience. A woman's selective response to elements of her reproductive context is centrally influenced by her earlier and current interactions with her mother and other pregnant and mothering women. In particular, an adolescent girl's relations with her mother influence the private meaning of her body and the way in which she experiences it. A major change in her perception of boundaries begins with menarche, a predictable pattern established by the monthly flow of blood. Menarche is a culturally ratified indication of a private, invisible, "deep" process. The change is confirmed in the first coital interaction, when a male body enters her own, and is socially and culturally integrated by pregnancy and the delivery of the first child. The irrevocable demonstration of a passage hitherto concealed from public acknowledgment, can mark the loss of a protective integument. Or it can contribute to a perception of boundaries characterized less by protectiveness than by interaction and participation with others, giving, and receiving, boundaries that tie a woman to her community rather than separating her from it.

The meaning of the change is elaborated when the young woman experiences her newly menstruating, reproductively capable, and potentially nurturing adult female body as desired, valued, or supported by identification with mother and positive sexual experience; or as dirty, shameful, or frightening, representing a status forbidden by mother. She may "live" her body (cf. Merleau-Ponty, 1942) as valued, affirming, and integrating, or as devalued or punished. Experiencing the "lived" adult female self may symbolize realization and unity, or destruction and displacement of the prohibiting mother from whom one has come.

Pregnancy is a time when the relationship with a mother can be re-created. To the degree that the prohibiting mother has been internalized ambivalently, the woman having intercourse without contraception, living through pregnancy and delivery and finally becoming a mother herself, experiences these events as negative. To the degree that they mean overcoming the mother's prohibitions and involve her symbolic displacement, they risk being self-destructive as well. Self-protection may require denial and repression, allowing her to abdicate responsibility for fertility behavior consequently experienced as passive and affectively flat or neutral.

The early exercise of volition in reproductive behavior may be a harbinger of later efforts at autonomy and self-determination. Making decisions is severely impeded by lack of information. The availability, source, quality, and timing of received sexual-reproductive information seem, despite the public media, a corollary to familial relationships, particularly to the mother's willingness to communicate openly and freely with her daughter. The daughter may initiate communication and may herself obtain information from maternal or other sources, but the capacity to initiate is itself a function of growing up. Lack of information, reflecting a lack of intimacy with one's mother, can lead to experiencing menarche as a surprising and shocking event, to be labeled ever after in the stark terms of its first appearance: "I saw the blood."

First coitus has private symbolic and symptomatic meanings when it constitutes a sought-after and successful attempt at conflict resolution, or personal integration. It also has meaning as a rite of passage marking the transition from girlhood to adulthood. The fact that intercourse has occurred is known not only to the woman and her first partner, but also often to her peers, relatives, and others if it is immediately succeeded by her first conjugal union and first pregnancy. For working-class women in Kingston, first coitus appears to be a type of private affirmation of self that does not necessarily include the sexual partner except instrumentally.

Contraceptive use or nonuse involves even more intentionality and a greater degree of communication with one's partner. Communication is, of course, more essential for the use of coitus-dependent methods, such as a condom or foam, than for an IUD or a pill, taken at a temporal, spatial, and emotional distance from the coital situation. Unilateral contraception may require the highest degree of intentionality and autonomy. The personal experience of contraception differs not only in method but also in its symbolic and interactive context.

Shared Private Conflict as an Aspect of Public Context

If a person grows up in a context engendering conflict about sexuality or reproduction, his or her sexual or reproductive behavior will reflect both the elements of conflict, however disguised, and attempts to solve it. If conflict exists in a sufficient number of people growing up in a particular context, their individual, repetitive attempts at solution, conscious or unconscious, will appear as a group pattern. Awareness that a particular way of behaving is expected even though it is not totally acceptable increases the likelihood that a person will behave in such a manner and decreases the likelihood that it will be experienced or

viewed as alien. If having several concurrent mates or more children than one can care for, for example, are regular occurrences
in a society, these behaviors may not be identified as problem-
atical either by oneself or by others. If they are expected, these
behaviors may assume a stereotypical or ritual quality with their
own social reinforcers, reducing the likelihood of conscious confrontation with their private determinants.

Other group patterns permit a person to express or gratify personally unacceptable aims without consciously confronting them.
Conflict resolution is facilitated and increased personal integration achieved, though at some cost, through acts that are socially
approved yet symptomatic. Such symptomatic acts may also arise
in response to a crisis. If male partners regularly disappear
shortly before the expected birth of first babies, for example, the
symptomatic, maladaptive response to such an event may also
constitute a group pattern.

The Sexual-Reproductive Scenario

The men and women interviewed for this study revealed a high
level of sexual activity resulting in many children. The men, 84
percent of whom were already fathers, appeared to be contracepting without conflict, utilizing the condom, which does not
require the woman's participation. Approximately one-fourth of
their primary mates, however, continued to use their own contraceptive as well—probably because of their uncertainty about the
man's reliability. Furthermore, the great majority of men had
additional visiting unions with women with whom they had frequent sexual intercourse. The number of women whom they regularly exposed to the possibility of insemination, and their past
history of ineffective contraception, make it difficult to be certain
that their current contraceptive use was in fact accompanied by
a continuing avoidance of fatherhood.

The sexual-reproductive careers of the women had almost
ritualistic scenarios. Menarche was unexpected and often shocking, experienced with shame. First coitus was often the consequence of male aggression, yet was frequently experienced as
just having "happened," without obvious reason. Usually it oc-

curred without contraception. Failure to contracept was unexplained or attributed to lack of knowledge despite general recognition of the availability of family planning advice and materials. For most it was soon followed by first pregnancy, while the girl was still in midadolescence. This demonstration of culturally valued fertility, a private experience with public significance, may also have unconscious symptomatic significance. Dismay at missing one's period despite behavior calculated to ensure its disappearance seems to follow the cultural script. So does the acute flare-up of maternal anger with its frequent threats of expulsion from the home. Both are temporary and are followed by acceptance of the new situation. The experience and attitude of the new grandmother are uncertain. About three-fourths of the new mothers, however, were unequivocally proud, happy, and pleased, and having the first baby appeared to be an integrative, conflict-resolving experience despite its potentially maladaptive consequences.

Freedom to act outside the scenario becomes possible with better education and a comparatively open relationship with one's mother that permits the early exchange of sexual-reproductive information. These conditions probably permit both a relatively unambivalent identification with the mother, who is not perceived as prohibiting the achievement of adult reproductive female status, and acquisition of a more tolerant and egalitarian view of males as fellow humans. Such women are least tied to the local "culture of motherhood" with its stereotyped views of men and domestic arrangements that entail the centrality of grandmothers and dependence by women upon their adult daughters for companionship and emotional support in old age. They are relatively free from the ritual, symptomatic compulsion to achieve womanhood and displace their mothers by early intercourse leading to early pregnancy. They are secure enough to have a first coital partner with whom they can talk, and are active, knowledgeable, and self-confident enough to contracept when they do have intercourse. Yet there are many points at which later events may negate the value of education, an open relationship with mother, and a later age of first coitus with good communication with the first partner. These are most clearly seen in women who did not form initial unions until age 21 or 22 but whose partners then broke their promises to marry them, emigrated and did not keep their promises to send for them, or concealed previous mates and children. In the period of loneliness —often combined with feelings of worthlessness—after the unexpected desertion there was sometimes a period of celibacy. Later liaisons were often formed with men of less education and apparent integrity than the first. The woman abandoned her initial resolve to contracept or delay pregnancy until she had a more stable conjugal union. Only rarely was anger a prominent feature. One still felt, five years, two mates, and two children later, that her first mate had so hurt her that she would "take a machete to him." Most, however, in their pain and disillusionment seemed to have lost their earlier alertness and optimism.

Successive pregnancies are less welcome than the first, especially to women without money or conjugal security. They seem most likely to occur at the disappearance of old mates and at the formation of new unions. The production of new—and now much more ambivalently desired—babies for new partners begins the repetitive reenactment of a drama with inherently contradictory ends. Intercourse as an essential part of forming a new alliance, relieving isolation, or hastening the eradication of subjective remnants of the old union, has some aspects of crisis resolution. Failure to contracept during coitus, "taking a chance" or simply "not thinking that it could happen," or rarely and consciously aiming for pregnancy extends the moment of crisis resolution into the continuing scenario. It is then played out through the next missed menstrual period, the subjective experience of pregnancy (which now less often includes desertion by the partner), and finally delivery, "calling for" the new baby and seeing it. An overt aim, formulated with the missed period—perhaps after a phase of chagrin or regret—is to symbolize, celebrate, and solidify the new union. It is she, the woman, who does this "for" the man by giving him a baby, sometimes his first, that presumably he desires. More accurately, perhaps, she confers on him the status of fatherhood, and the gift is a demonstration of his potency, fertility, and power. But the act is also a step in the direction of another aim, culturally supported and stimulated by the first expectations of later insecurity. This aim is the construction of her own family through the accumulation of children, leading to the day when—now in a leading familial position—she can function without an adult male in a context of her own making. The first aim is conscious. The second may be on the edge of awareness, accessible to introspection with help, but kept from the focus of attention by its implications: that she must take care of herself and her children and not depend on others except her maternal relatives. Having the baby and banding together with female relatives are more culturally congruent efforts to maintain a sense of integrity and worth than preventing conception by technological means. Paradoxically, the gift of a baby "for" the man can begin a process of converting him to an "outsider," for with the accumulation of children his functions, almost exclusively procreative, become superfluous. If he is unable or unwilling to function as an economic provider, he has no role.

None of our respondents spoke of "our" baby, or "we" had or are going to have a baby, or "he gave me" a baby. "Having a baby for him" connotes "having a baby without his participation" and giving it to him, but not permanently and only in symbolic form.

The woman least apt to be caught up in this sexual-reproductive drama is educated, urban, and modern. She values her capacity for self-determination outside the confines of biology. The ritual actors are in their way self-determining, but within the biological confines. They live their bodies in the traditional way. In contrast, those who manage themselves and their environments by using technical contraception live their bodies in a manner transcending biological imperatives. They can have at the onset of reproductive maturity the freedom that is only approximated by others toward the end of maturity. The woman who acts within the scenario seems obliged to go through each repetition until she reaches a point at which the next act is no longer required. Either her current male partner remains with her and both of their desires for new children are satisfied, she remains without a partner, or she enters a union in which, because of her own age and that of her new partner, sex and reproduction are no longer central issues. In the last case, because she will remain in close touch with her children and the man's offspring will be with their own mothers, he will have only peripheral emotional significance in the household. Or regardless of mate, the number of children she has produced may finally suffice for her own needs. Or the burden of increasing family size and the fatigue of repeated pregnancies will force her to use some form of birth control in the interest of personal survival. If she decides to pursue the definitive step of having herself sterilized, she may have to resist the (male) medical subculture of the island. As the drama for one short generation draws to an end, the new actors, already enculturated and trained, begin their own performance.

A Public Reproductive Policy

Public policy refers to government decisions intended to influence private behavior in a manner regarded desirable by official planners. It is rarely recognized by most citizens except in connection with specific issues or dramatic situations, as when the U.S. government in the late 1970s began to limit the use of public funds to support abortion. As most policies accumulate over generations and are embedded in the matrix of everyday life, they affect social structure and culture unnoticed, but with consequences for individuals not predictable from their legislative, executive, or judicial origins.

Population is a concern of public health and social policy, unique in that it touches upon such vital, personally and culturally protected areas as sexual interaction, childbearing, and child rearing. Jamaican fertility policy aims to reduce the rate of population growth through deferred first pregnancy, spaced births, and smaller families. These aims have obvious significance for the quality of life and competence of this generation and the next. The government has been vigorous in the provision of facilities and its efforts to make them known. Few major streets in Kingston are without a billboard telling people that pregnancy is not inevitable. The *Daily Gleaner* regularly advertises family planning services. After the data on this study had been gathered, large photographs of a handsome, seemingly nude, man urged the use of a new condom, the "Panther." The advertisers concluded that policy should be implemented in some ways congruent with the culture—contraceptive use in a setting in which male potency is important may be more acceptable if it is linked to the image of virility and sexual pleasure rather than to self-restraint, guilt, and medical care.

The views that policy makers consider important to national well-being, however, may not always be shared or even understood by the population they hope to influence. This is especially true when the behavior in question is private, affectively charged, conflictful, and involves strongly held cultural values. Reproductive behavior may be described in all of these ways. It is widely regarded as natural and as a human right not legitimately subject to regulation by others. Overt attempts to constrain it by governments, institutions, or individuals are often met with anger and fear. On the other hand, the idea of regulating one's fertility is not totally alien to Jamaicans or other peoples. Effective fertility control in the absence of coercion usually comes from individuals and couples concluding, on the basis of personal experience, that their own well-being will be furthered if they have fewer children. In this sense, through the exercise of their symbolic capacity they free themselves from domination by biological processes leading to unwanted reproduction. One of the most impressive demonstrations of the deliberate management of personal fertility, in an era preceding development of present-day contraceptive technology, was by U.S. women born between 1901 and 1910 (Dawson, Meny, and Ridley, 1980). Seventy-one percent in a survey of white, ever-married women in these cohorts practiced contraception, particularly those born between 1906 and 1910 who reached their peak reproductive years during the Great Depression. They used it to space their children as well as to terminate childbearing, and by so doing achieved the lowest average completed family size of any cohort since. By age 50 approximately 42 percent of them had had fewer than two children: 20

percent were childless and 22 percent had had only one child. These were mainly college-educated, urban, white-collar and non-Catholic. The most frequently used method was the condom (54.1 percent), followed by contraceptive douche (46.9 percent) and withdrawal (44.7 percent). From our point of view the most striking feature of these results is the implied degree of communication between mates. Successful use of the condom, and especially of withdrawal, require significant communication between mates. They also require a major commitment by the male partner to preventing the reproductive consequences of sexual intercourse, even at the expense of his personal pleasure. From the viewpoint of applying behavioral science data to public policy it is equally striking that the research reporting these findings mentions neither couple communication nor agreement as a possible reason for contraceptive success.

Culture undoubtedly constrains the policy approach to the vital issue of communication between couples. It is difficult to deal with couple communication as a public health concern in a society in which unions are typically unstable, men may impregnate a number of women without social penalty, and working-class households often center around two or three generations of women and their children. The "couple," a pair with a lifetime investment in each other, often does not exist in Jamaica until the woman's reproductive period is drawing to a close. It is difficult, also, to increase the effective sexual knowledge of adolescents in a culture overtly dominated by Victorian moral traditions that seem to function as an ideal, distracting attention from the realities of sexual-reproductive life. Implementing sex education, or "family life education," in the schools has been discussed at length by governmental and private groups. But progress has been minimal because of the scarcity of competent and comfortable instructors and the culturally and politically disturbing nature of the subject.

In addition to being culturally influenced, fertility-related behavior remains inseparable from the influence of a range of health and economic policies that affect job opportunities, couple interaction, and (through food prices as well as family structure) early developmental experience. Maternal nutrition influencing infant health reflects financial and emotional support from the sexual partner, the availability of food, and culturally determined preferences. Infectious illness reflects socioeconomically and culturally determined exposure and susceptibility to socially influenced patterns of endemic disease. Knoblock and Pasamanick's (1966) concept of a "cycle of reproductive casualty" is relevant here. They estimated that poverty-related deprivation, injuries, and illness of mother, fetus, or infant accounted in the early 1960s for approximately 20 percent of the institutionalized population of the United States.

The effect of disease on personal behavior and life experience is also determined by the treatment modes and institutions of a society, a function of its national health policy and its level of social and industrial development. But access to available institutions for treatment is also limited by ethnocentric attitudes toward health and treatment associated with minority group membership (Suchman, 1965), familial misinterpretation of symptomatic behavior as adaptive (Brody et al., 1967), lack of knowledge about gaining admission to healing institutions, and simple lack of money.

Public policy, then, is a pervasive though often unidentified influence upon the context of behavior. It contributes its own meaning to the expression of private aims and needs. In its overt and visible aspects it may influence a context's interactive features by designating particular acts, such as having several children, undesirable. It may modify the symbolic significance of having sexual intercourse, becoming pregnant, caring for babies, or forming a family. At the same time the covert, less visible aspects of policy (which may in fact be unenunciated) may vitiate the effect of the overt policy. Thus, public actions that indirectly tend to perpetuate poverty, unemployment, and low self-esteem reduce the effectiveness of policies directly intended to reduce fertility.

Reproductive Policy and the Culture of Jamaica

The official family planning message embodies the implicit and false assumptions that nuclear families are the island mode, that men and women communicate fully with each other, and that they regulate their sexual behavior on the basis of its anticipated consequences. It ignores the fact that mothers who were themselves impregnated early and have had several partners still raise their daughters with a "strictness" that deprives them of knowledge about reproductive development. This produces the kind of anger which, inadmissible to consciousness, is translated into disguised, symbolic action. Girls who lack the protection of older male relatives remain vulnerable to the casual sexual approaches of men who may utilize them to meet their own needs. They act on their wishes for experience and affirm themselves as adult females through sex and reproduction. Early intercourse and pregnancy (which for many foreclose later options) can also reflect ambivalent identification with mothers. Especially for adolescent girls indoctrinated with traditional matricentric values, reproduction represents not only hostility to their mother but also continued participation in a "culture of motherhood." The central value of this culture is the production of children without full, conscious, affective acceptance of male participation; this attitude of exclusion is most evident in the later pregnancies of women committed, after an early reproductive initiation, to an extended career in the roles of mother and grandmother. These women accept, while resenting male lack of support, the roles of both parents in child rearing.

The Jamaican sexual, reproductive, and household context, except for the availability of technical contraceptive methods, has not changed significantly in the last quarter-century. It has been described repeatedly (Kerr, 1952; Clarke, 1957). Its self-generating and self-perpetuating nature was emphasized by Blake (1961) on the basis of a three-month observation period in 1953-54. Yet changes are occurring. While younger respondents did not know significantly more about reproduction and contraception than the older ones, none revealed the total lack of knowledge reported in some earlier studies. Despite the prevalence of functional illiteracy, unemployment, substandard housing, and cultural isolation Jamaicans will inevitably acquire the attitudes, values, and perceptual and problem-solving styles of a technological civilization. As their consciousness changes so will their preconscious fantasies and ways of dealing with guilt or anxiety and resolving unconscious conflict. Their capacity for imagination and creative projection of themselves into the future will continue to grow. Conditions previously attributed to an unalterable fate will come to be perceived as susceptible to control through individual volition and action. With this possibility life assumes a different meaning; people begin to apprehend and test reality in different ways. But the process moves unevenly. The subgroup of respondents least affectively involved in their urban surroundings excluded dreams and fantasy from consciousness, saw more depressed and powerless figures in pictures, and held most tenaciously to traditional matricentric beliefs. They were, in a sense, cultural laggards. They had more children by more men in less stable unions than the others.

On the other hand, those who were best educated, occupationally advanced, and urban tended to have more stable conjugal unions and smaller families. Even so, these changes are not yet reflected in overall population statistics. Nor can they be confidently related to the official family planning campaign. In Jamaica, as elsewhere in the less industrialized world and in less advantaged segments of many industrial countries, men and women having little else over generations of blocked upward mobility and scarce resources still perceive parental status as a symbol of virility, self-worth, and community esteem. Children are objects that are truly and indubitably theirs. They provide meaningful life careers for women without alternative sources of fulfillment, measures of achievement for men without full-time or satisfying work, companionship in early life, and promise— though less securely than in the past—old-age security in the absence of other support. Beyond these benefits is a possibly perseverative need to produce sufficient offspring to survive to adulthood, despite significant decreases in infant mortality during the past generation. Nevertheless, the question remains how —given the continuing cultural value of parenthood, the still rigid system of rearing daughters, the apparently entrenched sexual-reproductive pattern, and the persistent poverty of the nation (Beckford, 1972)—public policy might create a new situation, one in which people would voluntarily have fewer children, for whom they could care more adequately, and who would subsequently have a better chance for satisfying lives for themselves and their own children. This question requires attention to historically conditioned social structure as well as to more personally immediate psychosocial considerations.

Public Policy for Family Stability and Communication

The Conjugal Union

The most salient features of the lower-class Jamaican reproductive context are the adolescent onset of sexual partnerships whose instability eventually leads to multiple pregnancies and impregnators, and, for children, the absence of a consistent, supportive father. A group of women interviewed after delivery of their second or later child in Kingston's largest public maternity hospital included only 4 percent who were legally married to the new "baby-father." The trend revealed in our data and those from the maternity hospital (table 14) fits the union status of 299 women who had discontinued attendance at family planning clinics in 1969 (Bracken, 1976). Of these, 70.6 percent were unattached or in a visiting status at the time of their first pregnancy, 23 percent were in common-law unions, and 6.4 percent were legally married.

The 1970 census (table 16) suggests a more stable context, with more respondents married than in any other category, followed by unmarried cohabiting and then a variety of visiting or broken unions. But if to the visiting and broken unions are added women listed as never having been in a union, the number approaches or surpasses those in the married category, depending upon age. Approximately one-third of women aged 15-44 islandwide are listed as never having had a husband or regular sexual partner. Furthermore, the census figures include a much larger representation of older women, especially those past reproductive age and from rural communities more socially integrated than Kingston. Of 22,473 women between ages 15 and 44 residing in Kingston Parish only 10.2 percent were legally married. This contrasts with almost 28 percent of 86,286 St. Andrew respondents (Census, vol. 8, 1976). With age, and especially past the point of child-bearing and rearing, visiting relationships tend to terminate. More women have relatively permanent, common-law or married cohabiting mates, and the rest remain solitary. Of 8,169 Kingston Parish women aged 45-64, 31.5 percent are married. Almost one-fourth still have never had a regular partner. Except for a very few who remain in visiting status the rest are equally divided between common-law cohabiting relationships and living alone after having separated from their partners. In the more stable rural St. Andrew part of the KMA almost half the 45-to-64-year-old women are married, and correspondingly fewer, approximately 15 percent, remain single.

Islandwide figures are similar. There is a gradual increase in the number of married women up to age 35-39, a relative plateau between ages 40 and 49, and a decline, possibly due to mortality, thereafter. Women who are contracepting or having babies tend to do so before the age when unions become institutionalized, whether by law or shared residence. Visiting relationships are most prevalent between ages 15 and 24. Common-law cohabiting unions peak between ages 20 and 29, with subsequent reductions as people enter legal marriage. The erosion of early unions begins at about the same time, so the number of women separated from common-law mates rises sharply between ages 20 and 24. The increase in married women living separately from their husbands is more gradual, becoming visible in statistics by age 25 but not leveling off until ages 50 to 54. Legalizing the union may offer some protection against its dissolution in a society of late marriages preceded by a diversity of partners, in contrast with one in which marriage to an early partner is the norm.

Although many women aged 20-24 at the time of the 1970 census had had their entire sexual-reproductive careers in the era of the government contraceptive campaign, and family planning services had been available for years, relatively few had not been pregnant. The incidence of pregnancy is highest for those in unstable relationships. More of the legally married (17.7 percent), who presumably had the most constant sexual exposure, had no children at all. Less than 10 percent of unmarried cohabitors and no woman in a visiting union had avoided pregnancy. Either the married women had had less intercourse than the others or they have contracepted more regularly and effectively. Or, conversely, the unmarried, especially those who did not live together, had had more intercourse or, in response to pressure from their mates to "have a baby for" them, they did not use contraceptives. Figures for those with three or more children indicate the same trend for greater fertility among the unmarried, although this is less marked for women in visiting than common-law unions.

Between ages 30-34, with more exposure to sexual intercourse the trend is more marked. Whereas a residual of approximately 7 percent childlessness persists among the cohabitors (married or common-law), the proportion of women with three or more children rises with less institutionalized conjugal status: 62.4 percent for the married, 76.5 percent for the cohabiting, and 87.3 percent for the visiting, none of whom are childless. No woman still in visiting status by age 40-44 has not had children, and 91.8 percent have had three or more, approximately 20 percent more than those who live together.

The widespread multiple mating, serial and concurrent, fits the male deficit pattern; that is, in order for most women to have the experiences of coitus and pregnancy, most men must have intercourse with and impregnate more than one woman. National statistics confirm the impression from our samples that most women in less stable unions become pregnant and that *union instability is positively related to high reproductive performance.* Within our population of condom-using men those of highest status had multiple sexual partners, but these were concurrent and did not result in pregnancies. On the other hand, the lower-status men, who tended to be older (and currently cohabiting with fewer concurrent partners), had not been regular contraceptive users, embraced traditional male-dominant values, and had produced more children with serial partners in their younger, pre-cohabiting years.

These data do not fit a prediction from the precontraceptive era (Blake, 1961, pp. 249-250) that stabilization of "lower-class Jamaican sexual associations," with more sexual exposure for the female partner, would increase the island's fertility by at least 30 percent. It seems, on the contrary, that the amount of sexual exposure is less central in determining individual fertility than the quality of the relationship between mates. A man and woman in a stable union who can communicate with each other on an affectively meaningful level and have some commitment to a shared future can negotiate the matter of producing children and using or not using contraception. Joint and explicit decision making is possible. A lower-class woman with a mate with whom she does not communicate must make a unilateral decision to contracept or risk offending him or precipitating a quarrel by proposing contraception (Brody, Ottey, and LaGranade, 1974). Or—because she has no other assurance of stability—she may try to hold him by acceding to his request "to have a baby for him." These conclusions fit data reported in the late 1950s, when there were only two family planning clinics in Jamaica. New knowledge alone was not accompanied by an increase in a woman's actual contraceptive use. The crucial corollary of increased contraceptive use was an increase in the level of communication between sexual partners (Stycos and Back, 1964).

The Family of Origin and Induced Cultural Change

The indications are strong that first pregnancy in Jamaica may represent not only the adolescent girl's acquiescence to her partner's request and a possible attempt to tie him to her but also participation in a socially transmitted pattern reinforced by the high value accorded to motherhood. Early first intercourse and pregnancy, leading to continued low contraceptive and high reproductive performance associated with high partner diversity, are associated with beliefs implying the centrality of mothers and a peripheral status for fathers. These include a traditional view of grandmother, the belief in a predetermined "lot" of babies, and the idea that a woman's primary responsibility is to her mother rather than to her mate. They are part of a complex including lack of maternal information and poor communication with the first partner. In this context the woman, regardless of conscious rationalizations, may have her baby at a more fundamental, unconscious or covert level "for" herself as part of the female tradition, rather than for the man. With increasing age and disillusionment with men the production of children to satisfy personal needs and provide a support system—despite the pain and problems of inadequate economic resources—becomes more explicit. The prevalence of exclusively female households among the women respondents suggests the context in which these beliefs and attitudes develop and are emphasized.

Beyond these considerations the exact proportion of Jamaican births accounted for by women in unstable associations is not known. It cannot be assumed, therefore, that their transfer into more permanent unions would result in higher national fertility (Marino, 1970). Nor, given the deficit in the number of males, can it be assumed that a shift toward conjugal stability would not result in a significant decrease in the number of total unions. It may plausibly be argued that a trend to conjugal stability would, on the contrary, result in an increase of unmated, childless women. This increase would not be offset by increased fertility of those more stably mated, because greater stability would probably be accompanied by increases in the age of first coitus and union formation and increased communication about and use of contraception.

Our findings suggest that greater conjugal stability accompanied by more open communication between couples is essential to lowering individual reproductive performance and thus to reducing family size and eventually the rate of population growth. A relatively small population of males, more educated and occupationally advanced than the bulk of the population, regularly uses condoms and manages its fertility unilaterally. These men, unlike the majority of lower socioeconomic status, are sexually active without reproducing. If they can affirm their self-esteem through occupational achievement that may be impeded by the responsibilities of early fatherhood they will not produce children until they can comfortably support them.

Strengthening the family is a cultural process that public policy action can facilitate. Public policy in such a case would deliberately aim at changing the sexual-reproductive culture of the society. Whether imposing legal penalties might be a way of ensuring paternal responsibility is a question that has been raised, but it is a difficult one. Incentives may be more effective. Social legislation could reward the development of stable family units and the assumption of paternal responsibility. Possibilities range from government subsidies for housing based on applications by couples to specific forms of assistance for a man's first two children but not for later ones.

Nonlegislated approaches may be even more useful. Discussion groups for couples or educational groups for women that require the attendance of mates, for example, might help develop a context in which such participation will occur more easily. Sex education seems essential for both boys and girls prior to puberty (Brody, Ottey, and LaGranade, 1976), including attention to the importance of intimacy in sexual relations and the exploitation of sex as a means of gaining personal power and self-esteem. In the absence of stable family units or free communication between mother and child, implementing sex education will require training schoolteachers who are not only technically competent but also emotionally comfortable with the subject. It should decrease the need of females to utilize men in the expression of anger against their mothers and to demonstrate to themselves their own independent fertility. At the same time attention needs to be given to the generally neglected relations between mother and son. Although our data for this relationship are only anecdotal they suggest strongly that—in sharp contrast to the sexual discipline imposed upon girls—the mothers in these essentially fatherless homes are extremely permissive with their sons and may implicitly tolerate the development of attitudes leading to procreatively irresponsible behavior.

The alleged or perceived social and economic advantages of having several children require systematic attention. Although the threat of social isolation in old age continues to be important, there are no reliable data on the social circumstances of older Jamaican men and women. Knowledge of the financial support and companionship provided older parents by their adult children is a prerequisite to the formulation of new social security policies. Such policies are an essential aspect of solving any "population problem."

Direct Family Planning Services

Personnel

The characteristics of family planning facilities, the training of their personnel, and the way in which services are provided are important determinants of their acceptability to the population to be served. Most of the elements making for congruence or its lack between voluntary family planning programs and the sociocultural context of Jamaicans are common to other not fully industrialized or modernized countries.

The "clinic" model of a family planning center has some advantages, but the symbolic (and to some degree actual) association of a clinic with physicians and illness discourages some potential clients. Furthermore, the ambivalence of many physicians toward definitive contraception and sterilization betrays a male-oriented attitude as well as one that at times seems both moralistic and compulsive.

The JFPA experiment in training country nanas in technical contraceptive methods is a logical approach to the problem of social and method acceptability. The obvious solution is to broaden and diversify the sources from which family planning advice and services may be obtained, and to integrate them more into the community, both spatially and interpersonally. Recruiting and educating older women as agents of social change might be a difficult but worthwhile approach. They command respect and attention and may be unusually effective if they can offer themselves as models of women becoming independent of biological forces and free from burdens imposed by men.

The selection and training of family planning workers should include particular attention to their private views and the degree to which deeply held values antithetical to personal fertility control might, without their awareness, impair their effectiveness as agents of social change. A variety of group process techniques, involving personal affective encounters and increased sensitivity to one's own private feelings and public messages as well as to those of others, may be useful in screening and training candidates. The fact that young noncohabiting women with few children—that is, those with fewest meaningful relationships—are most likely to discontinue contraceptive use confirms an impression that forming a family without a father is often a defense against feelings of low self-esteem and social isolation. Nonprofessional family planning workers who speak the language of the local community might provide an important source of identification to lonely young women. Support aiming at increased self-esteem and autonomy can increase willingness and ability to regulate one's biological as well as social destiny.

Counseling for Family Stability

Family planning in its most constructive sense also concerns the new parents' families of origin. Counseling both the newly pregnant girl and her mother can constitute the intervention essential for re-creating a relationship that will permit the new mother to become, herself, a more effective parent. The potential father and his relationships with his parents have been largely ignored. If family stability is to become a cornerstone of population policy, however, the attitudes of both the young father and his family of origin are crucial targets for systematic attention.

Contraceptive Methods

The folk healing context of working-class Jamaican life and the nature of the indigenous methods used in attempts to delay, space, or finally prevent more pregnancies suggest that certain method characteristics are more acceptable than others.

Most prominent is the desirability of a method that is "natural." It should, ideally, require no substance or device. A type of rhythm method would fit this model, but the required self-monitoring could be difficult for poor, illiterate people living under disadvantaged circumstances. Because no such fully natural method is as yet available, effective, and acceptable, how-

ever, certain characteristics of a substance used become important. It should be related to or extracted from one of the familiar
plants or trees on the island, or at least should be sufficiently
familiar to have a folk or colloquial designation. Devices such
as the IUD and oral contraceptives are perceived as powerful,
of foreign origin, unnatural, and therefore unpredictable and
potentially dangerous. They cannot be grown in one's back
yard, gathered "in the hills," discussed knowledgeably by older
women, or taken without the intervention of a group of strange,
technically trained people. These features all contain the threat
of uncontrollability. One approach would be to involve people in
the final steps of preparing the method. They could, for example,
obtain a powder and themselves boil it with water in order to
make it into a "tea."

Closely related are the matters of availability and privacy. A
person who obtains a natural substance, prolongs her own lactation, or simply abstains from coitus can do so without violating
her privacy or the expectations of her neighbors. A trip to a drugstore or family planning center, however close, requires a public
exhibition of intent and, furthermore, exposure to the inquiries of
strangers.

An acceptable method probably should not require vaginal
manipulation. In this sense a pill or injectable would be less disturbing than an IUD or diaphragm. In the Jamaican context a
"tea" or infusion would be experienced as the most natural.

The method should carry connotations of vitality and strength
rather than weakness or illness. It should therefore be obtainable
from nonmedical sources without requiring the intervention of
physicians or nurses, and should not be surrounded by the para-
phernalia of disease. Similarly, it should connote increased potency, virility, and potential fertility rather than the opposite; it
might, for example, be mixed or taken along with a substance
connoting potency, such as malt or stout. At any event, the presentation of the method could take this consideration into account.

Presentations should avoid any implication that the method will
permanently limit fertility. A more acceptable focus would be the
display of strength inherent in the capacity to manage oneself.

Advertisements depicting extra children as a sign of weakness or irresponsibility are apt to evoke guilt and despair, with a view of contraception as somehow remedial or expiatory rather than potency enhancing.

Finally, an acceptable method should not interfere with the regularity of the menstrual flow. It should rather ensure that a woman "sees her period."

Summary

Without doubt social modernization facilitates a population policy intended to reduce family size, encourage spacing of children, and slow overall population growth. As part of the movement toward cultural integrity modernization should help provide the shared symbols and values that permit popular identification with national purpose. Jamaica and other developing countries, however, may not be able to achieve modern status without a reduction in the rate of population increase. Public policy without coercion will thus require attention to private aims and conflicts and to shared cultural patterns. All these will influence not only the nature, advertisement, and presentation of family planning services but also the gradual development of an ethos favoring parent-child communication, sex education at puberty, increased autonomy for women, delayed first pregnancy, spaced births, small ultimate family size, and a reduction in passing children on to be reared by others. The promotion of stable conjugal unions with adequate communication between partners is essential to the achievement of these aims.

References

Alexander, J. 1976. A study of the cultural domain of "relatives." *American Ethnologist* 3:17-38.

Arnhoff, F. N. 1975. Social consequences of policy toward mental illness. *Science* 188:1277-81.

Asprey, G. F., and P. Thornton. 1953-1955. Medicinal plants of Jamaica: parts I, II, III, IV. *West Indian Medical Journal* 2:233-252; 3:17-41; 4:69-82, 145-168.

Baldwin, W., and V. Cain. 1980. The children of teenage parents. *Family Planning Perspectives* 12:34-43.

Barker, R. G. 1968. *Ecological Psychology.* Stanford: Stanford University Press.

Barrett, L. 1973. Portrait of a Jamaican healer: African medical lore in the Caribbean. *Caribbean Quarterly* 19:6-19.

Beckford, G. 1972. *Persistent poverty: underdevelopment in plantation economies of the Third World.* London: Oxford University Press.

Beckwith, M. W. 1927. *Notes on Jamaican ethnobotany.* New York: Vassar College Folklore Foundation.

Bennett, J. W. 1976. Anticipation, adaptation, and the concept of culture in anthropology. *Science* 192:847-853.

Berger, P., B. Berger, and H. Kellner. 1974. *The homeless mind: modernization and consciousness.* New York: Random House, Vintage Books.

Black, C. 1973. *A new history of Jamaica.* London: Wm. Collins and Sangster.

Blake, J. *Family structure in Jamaica.* 1961. New York: Free Press.

Boas, F. 1940. In *Freedom: its meaning,* ed. R. N. Anshen. New York: Harcourt Brace.

Bongaarts, J. 1980. Does malnutrition affect fecundity? A summary of evidence. *Science* 208:564-569.

Bracken, M. B. 1976. Contraception and pregnancy after dropping out of family planning clinics: a national interview survey in Jamaica. *Social Biology* 23:55-65.

Braithwaite, E. 1970. *Folk culture of the slaves in Jamaica.* London: New Beacon Books.

Brodber, E. 1974. *Abandonment of children in Jamaica.* Mona, Jamaica: Institute of Social and Economic Research, University of the West Indies.

Brody, E. B. 1966. Cultural exclusion, character and illness. *American Journal of Psychiatry* 122:852-858.

———. 1968. Culture, symbol and value in the social etiology of behavioral deviance. In *Social Psychiatry*, ed. J. Zubin, pp. 8-23. New York: Grune & Stratton.

———. 1973. *The lost ones: social forces and mental illness in Rio de Janeiro.* New York: International Universities Press.

———. 1974. Psychocultural aspects of contraceptive behavior in Jamaica. *Journal of Nervous and Mental Disease* 159:108-119.

———. 1976. Reproductive freedom, coercion, and justice: some ethical aspects of population policy and practice. *Social Science and Medicine* 10:553-557.

———, ed. 1970. *Behavior in new environments: adaptation of migrant populations.* Beverly Hills: Sage.

Brody, E. B., R. L. Derbyshire, and C. Schleifer. 1967. How the young adult Baltimore negro male becomes a mental hospital statistic. In *Psychiatric epidemiology and mental health planning*, ed. R. R. Monroe, G. D. Klee, and E. B. Brody, pp. 206-219. American Psychiatric Association Research Reports, no. 22. Washington, D.C.

Brody, E. B., and L. F. Newman. 1981. Ethnography and psychoanalysis: comparative ways of knowing. *Journal of the American Academy of Psychoanalysis* 9:17-32.

Brody, E. B., F. Ottey, and J. LaGranade. 1974. Couple communication in the contraceptive decision making of Jamaican women. *Journal of Nervous and Mental Disease* 159:407-412.

———. 1976. Early sex education in relationship to later coital and reproductive behavior: evidence from Jamaican women. *American Journal of Psychiatry* 133:969-972.

Brookings Bulletin. 1980. 16 (3):14-15.

Campbell, S. 1974a. Folklore and food habits. *Jamaica Journal* 8:56-59.

———. 1974b. Bush teas, a cure-all. *Jamaica Journal* 8:60-65.

Card, J., and L. Wise. 1978. Teenage mothers and teenage fathers: the impact of early childbearing on the parents' personal and professional lives. *Family Planning Perspectives* 10:199-205.

Clarke, E. 1953. Land tenure and the family in four communities in Jamaica. *Social and Economic Studies* 1:81-118.

————. 1966. *My mother who fathered me.* 2nd ed. London: Allen and Unwin.

Cohen, Y. A. 1955. Four categories of interpersonal relationships in the family and community in a Jamaican village. *Anthropology Quarterly* 3:121-147.

Cronon, E. 1969. *Black Moses: the story of Marcus Garvey.* 2nd ed. Madison: University of Wisconsin Press.

Cumper, G. E. 1956. Population movements in Jamaica, 1830-1950. *Social and Economic Studies* 5:261-280.

————. 1963. Preliminary analysis of population growth and social characteristics in Jamaica, 1943-1960. *Social and Economic Studies* 12:394-431.

Curtin, P. 1955. *Two Jamaicas.* Cambridge, Mass.: Harvard University Press.

Dawson, D. A., D. J. Meny, and J. D. Ridley, 1980. Fertility control in the United States before the contraceptive revolution. *Family Planning Perspectives* 12:76-86.

DeCharms, R. 1968. *Personal causation: the internal affective determinants of behavior.* New York: Academic Press.

Digest of Family Planning Perspectives. 1980. 12:108-110.

Douglas, M. 1978. *Purity and danger.* 2nd ed. London: Routledge and Kegan Paul.

Dunnell, K. 1979. *Family formation, 1976.* London: Office of Population Censuses and Surveys, Social Survey Division, Her Majesty's Stationery Office.

Durant-Gonzalez, V. 1976. Role and status of rural Jamaican women: higglering and mothering. Ph.D. diss., University of California at Berkeley.

Elkins, W. F. 1969. Black power in the British West Indies: the Trinidad longshoremen's strike of 1919. *Science and Society* 33:71-75.

Elster, A., and E. McAnarney. 1980. Medical and psychosocial risks of pregnancy and childbearing during adolescence. *Pediatric Annals* 9:13-20.

Eyre, L. A. 1972a. *Geographic aspects of population dynamics in Jamaica.* Boca Raton: Florida Atlantic University Press.

————. 1972b. The shantytowns of Montego Bay, Jamaica. *Geographical Review* 62:394-413.

————. 1979. Quasi-urban melange settlement: cases from St. Catherine and St. James, Jamaica. *Geographical Review* 69:95-100.

Fawcett, J. T., and M. H. Bornstein. 1973. Modernization, individual modernity and fertility. In *Psychological perspectives on population*, ed. J. T. Fawcett, pp. 106-134. New York: Basic Books.

Figueroa, J. 1971. *Society, schools and progress in the West Indies*. Oxford: Pergamon Press.

Floyd, B. 1970. Rural land development in Jamaica. *Area* 1:7-11.

Francis, S. 1973. Social welfare aspects of family planning. Unpublished manuscript. Cited by V. Durant-Gonzalez, 1976.

Frazier, E. F. 1957. *The negro family in the United States*. Rev. ed. New York: Macmillan.

Furstenberg, F. 1976a. *Unplanned parenthood: the social consequences of teenage childbearing*. New York: Macmillan.

————. 1976b. The social consequences of teenage parenthood. *Family Planning Perspectives* 8:148-164.

Garland, S., and R. Trudeau. 1972. Population policy research: a critique and an alternative. In *Research in the politics of population*, ed. R. L. Clinton and R. K. Godwin, pp. 17-39. Lexington, Mass.: Lexington Books.

Gentles, N. H. 1968. A case of Jones Town: an analysis of population movement with the Kingston metropolitan area. Bachelor's thesis, Department of Geography, University of the West Indies, Kingston.

Goffman, E. 1957. The characteristics of total institutions. *Symposium on Preventive and Social Psychiatry*. Washington, D.C.: U.S. Government Printing Office.

Gonzalez, N. 1969. *Black Carib household structure*. Seattle: University of Washington Press.

Goody, E. N. 1975. Delegation of parental roles in West Africa and the West Indies. In *Socialization and communication in primary groups*, ed. T. R. Williams, pp. 125-158. The Hague: Mouton.

Henriques, F. 1953. *Family and colour in Jamaica*. London: Eyre and Spottiswoode.

Herskovits, M. 1937. *Life in a Haitian valley*. New York: Alfred A. Knopf.

————. 1941. *The myth of the Negro past*. New York: Harper & Brothers.

————. 1946. Problem, method, and theory of Afro-American studies. *Phylon* 7:337-354.

————. 1948. *Man and his works.* New York: Alfred A. Knopf.

————. 1951. The present status and needs of Afro-American research. *Journal of Negro History* 36:123-147.

Huber, D. H., and A. R. Khan. 1979. Contraceptive distribution in Bangladesh villages: the initial impact. *Studies in Family Planning* 10:246-253.

Inkeles, A., and D. H. Smith. 1974. *Becoming modern.* Cambridge, Mass.: Harvard University Press.

Inkeles, S. 1969. Making men modern: on the causes and consequences of individual change in six developing countries. *American Journal of Sociology* 75:208-225.

Jamaican Information Service. 1970. *Facts on Jamaica.* JIS no. 1. Kingston.

————. 1972a. *The People of Jamaica.* JIS no. 3. Kingston.

————. 1972b. *Religion in Jamaica.* JIS no. 7. Kingston.

Jamaica Family Planning Association. 1971. *Annual Report, 1971.* St. Ann's Bay: Jamaica Family Planning Association.

Jamaica population census, 1970. 1973. Bulletin no. 1. Kingston: Division of Censuses and Surveys, Department of Statistics.

————. 1973. Bulletin no. 2. Kingston: Division of Censuses and Surveys, Department of Statistics.

————. 1974. Bulletin no. 3. Kingston: Division of Censuses and Surveys, Department of Statistics.

————. 1976. Bulletin no. 4. Kingston: Division of Censuses and Surveys, Department of Statistics.

————. 1976. Bulletin no. 5. Kingston: Division of Censuses and Surveys, Department of Statistics.

————. 1976. In *1970 Population Census of the Commonwealth Caribbean,* vol. 8, *Fertility.* Kingston: Census Research Programme, University of the West Indies.

Jekyll, W., ed. 1904. *Jamaican song and story.* Reprint, New York: Dover, 1966.

Keller, A. B., J. H. Sims, W. E. Henry, and T. J. Crawford. 1970. Psychological sources of "resistance" to family planning. *Merrill-Palmer Quarterly* 16:286-302.

Kerr, M. 1952. *Personality and conflict in Jamaica.* Liverpool: Liverpool University Press.

Klein, G. S. 1976. *Psychoanalytic theory: an exploration of essentials.* New York: International Universities Press.

Klerman, L., and J. Jekel. 1973. *School-age mothers: problems, pro-*

grams and policy. Hamden, Conn.: Shoe String Press.

Kluckhohn, C. 1944. *Mirror for man.* New York: McGraw-Hill.

Knobloch, H., and B. Pasamanick. 1966. Prospective studies on the epidemiology of reproductive casualty. *Merrill-Palmer Quarterly* 12: 127-143.

Kohn, M. 1969. *Class and conformity: a study in values.* Havenwood, Ill.: Dorsey Press.

————. 1973. Social classes: a critical review and a reformulation. *Schizophrenia Bulletin* 7:60-79.

Kubie, L. S. 1974. The drive to become both sexes. *Psychoanalytic Quarterly* 13:349-426.

Landman, J. P., et al. 1976. Breast feeding in decline in Kingston, Jamaica, 1973. *West Indian Medical Journal* 25(1):43-57.

LeVine, R. 1973. *Culture, behavior, and personality.* Chicago: Aldine Press.

Levy, R. 1973. *The Tahitians.* Chicago: University of Chicago Press.

Lewin, Olive. 1973. Forty folksongs of Jamaica. Washington, D.C.: General Secretariat of the Organization of American States.

Linton, R. 1945. *The cultural background of personality.* New York: Appleton-Century.

Long, J. 1971. Choice of medical practitioners in a developing area of Jamaica: dynamics of changing concepts of disease and its treatment. Paper presented to the American Anthropological Association, New York, November 1971.

Lowe, H. 1972. Folk medicine in Jamaica. *Jamaica Journal* 6:20-24.

Lowenthal, D. 1972. *West Indian societies.* London: Oxford University Press.

Marino, A. 1970. Family, fertility, and sex ratios in the British Caribbean. *Population Studies* 24 (2):159-172.

Marriott, J. 1968. Psychiatric symptomatology in Jamaican medical patients. *West Indian Medical Journal* 17:109-115.

McKay, D. M. 1964. Communication and meaning. In *Cross-cultural understanding: epistemology in anthropology,* ed. F. S. C. Northrop and H. H. Livingston, pp. 162-179. New York: Harper & Row.

Menken, J. Forthcoming. The health and demographic consequences of adolescent pregnancy and childbearing. In *Adolescent pregnancy and childbearing,* ed. C. Chilman. Washington, D.C.: U.S. Government Printing Office.

Merleau-Ponty, M. 1942. *The structure of behavior.* Reprint, Boston: Beacon Press, 1963.

Meuller, J. H., K. F. Schuessler, and H. L. Costner. 1970. *Statistical reasoning in sociology*. 2nd ed. Boston: Houghton Mifflin.

Miller, K. A., and A. Inkeles. 1974. Modernity and acceptance of family limitation in four developing countries. *Journal of Social Issues* 30:167-188.

Mintz, S. 1966. The Caribbean as a socio-culture area. *Journal of World History* 9:912-937.

Moore, J., and G. Simpson. 1957-1958. A comparative study of acculturation in Morant Bay and West Kingston, Jamaica. *Zaire* 11:979-1019 and 12:65-87.

Moore, K., and L. Waite. 1977. Early childbearing and educational attainment. *Family Planning Perspectives* 9:220-225.

National Center for Health Statistics. 1979. Natality statistics. *Monthly Vital Statistics Report* 27:11. Washington, D.C.: U.S. Government Printing Office.

National Family Planning Board. 1976. *Statistical report, June quarter, 1974*. Kingston.

National Planning Agency. 1972. *Economic Survey of Jamaica*. Kingston: Government of Jamaica.

———. 1978. *Urban growth and management study: final report*. Kingston: Government of Jamaica.

Netherlands Ministry of Foreign Affairs, Directorate for International Technical Assistance. 1968. Jamaica's Social Problems. Mimeographed.

Nettleford, R. 1970. *Mirror, mirror: identity, race and protest in Jamaica*. Jamaica: Wm. Collins and Sangster.

Newman, L. F. 1980. Non-prescriptive fertility regulating methods: report on a cross-cultural research project. In *Proceedings of the Fifth International Congress of Psychosomatic Obstetrics and Gynecology*. London: Academic Press.

Norris, K. 1962. *Search for identity*. London: Oxford University Press.

Norton, A. 1974. The growth (1942-1970) and residential structure (1968) of the Kingston metropolitan area. Mimeographed. Kingston: Department of Geography, University of the West Indies.

———. 1978. *Shanties and skyscrapers: growth and structure of modern Kingston*. Mona: Institute of Social and Economic Research, University of the West Indies.

O'Connell, M., and M. J. Moore. 1980. The legitimacy status of first births to U.S. women aged 15-24, 1939-1978. *Family Planning Perspectives* 12:16-25.

Pakistan Family Planning Council. 1973. *Pakistan impact survey.* Islamabad.

Park, R. E. 1950. *Race and culture.* Glencoe, Ill.: The Free Press.

Patterson, O. *The sociology of slavery.* 1967. Reprint, London: Granada Publishing.

Phillips, A. 1973. *Adolescence in Jamaica.* Kingston and London: Jamaican Publishing House and Macmillan.

Polanyi, M. *Personal knowledge.* 1958. London: Routledge and Kegan Paul. Reprint, 1973.

The Population Council. 1971. *Jamaica: country profiles.* New York.

Rawls, J. 1971. *A theory of justice.* Cambridge, Mass.: Harvard University Press.

Roberts, G. W. 1957. *The population of Jamaica.* Cambridge: Cambridge University Press.

————. 1973. *Provisional estimates of population movements in Jamaica to 1990.* Kingston: privately printed.

Rotter, J. B. 1966. Generalized expectancies for internal versus external control of reinforcement. *Psychological Monograph* 80 (1).

Ryder, N. B. 1959. Fertility. In *The study of population: an inventory and appraisal,* ed. P. M. Hauser and O. D. Duncan, pp. 400-436. Chicago: University of Chicago Press.

Sanderson, F., and S. Roy. 1979. India's food prospects and policies. Washington, D.C.: Brookings Institute.

Sapir, E. 1932. Cultural anthropology and psychology. *Journal of Abnormal and Social Psychology* 27:229-242.

Schutz, A. 1962. *The problem of social reality.* The Hague: Nijhoff.

Schneider, D. M., and R. T. Smith. 1973. *Class differences and sex roles in American kinship and family structure.* Englewood Cliffs, N. J.: Prentice-Hall.

Seaga, E. 1969. Revival cults in Jamaica. *Jamaica Journal* 3:3-13.

Second five year plan, 1970-75, vol. 4. Kingston: Central Planning Unit, Ministry of Finance and Planning.

Simpson, G. 1957. The nine-night ceremony in Jamaica. *Journal of American Folklore* 70:329-335.

————. 1970. *Religious cults of the Caribbean: Trinidad, Jamaica, and Haiti.* Rio Piedras, Puerto Rico: Institute of Caribbean Studies, University of Puerto Rico.

Sinclair, S. 1974. A fertility analysis of Jamaica: recent trends with reference to the parish of St. Ann. *Social and Economic Studies* 23:588-635.

Smith, K. A. 1971. Some socio-cultural and medical problems related to family planning in Jamaica, West Indies. Ph.D. diss., Yale University.

Smith, M. B. 1972. "Normality" for an abnormal age. In *Modern psychiatry and clinical research: essays in honor of Roy R. Grinker*, ed. D. Offer and D. X. Freedman, pp. 102-119. New York: Basic Books.

———. 1973. A social psychological view of fertility. In *Psychological perspectives on population*, ed. J. T. Fawcett, pp. 3-18. New York: Basic Books.

Smith, M. G. 1960. The African heritage in the Caribbean. In *Caribbean studies: a symposium*, ed. V. Rubin, pp. 34-46. 2nd ed. Seattle: University of Washington Press.

———. 1962. *West Indian family structure*. Seattle: University of Washington Press.

———. 1966. Introduction to *My mother who fathered me*, 2nd ed., by E. Clarke, pp. i-xliv. London: Allen and Unwin.

Smith, M. G., R. Augier, and R. Nettleford. 1960. *The Rastafari movement in Kingston, Jamaica*. Kingston: Institute of Social and Economic Research, University of the West Indies.

Stone, C. 1973. *Class, race, and political behavior in urban Jamaica.* Kingston: Institute of Social and Economic Research, University of the West Indies.

Stonequist, E. V. 1937. *The marginal man.* New York: Charles Scribner's and Sons.

Suchman, E. 1965. Social factors in medical deprivation. *American Journal of Public Health* 55:1725-71.

Stycos, J. M. 1965. Problems of fertility control in underdeveloped areas in the population crisis. In *The population crisis: implications and plans for action*, ed. L. Ng and S. Mudd, pp. 44-58. Bloomington: Indiana University Press.

Stycos, J. M., and K. W. Back. 1964. *The control of human fertility in Jamaica.* Ithaca: Cornell University Press.

Trussell, T. 1976. Economic consequences of teenage childbearing. *Family Planning Perspectives* 8:184.

United Nations. 1953. *The determinants and consequences of population trends: a summary of the findings of studies on the relationships between population changes and economic and social conditions.* Population Studies, no. 17. New York: United Nations.

———. 1969. Economic and Social Council. Resolution 1672 (LII). New York: United Nations.

————. 1971. Estimates of urban and rural populations by regions and counties, 1960-1985. *UN Monthly Bulletin of Statistics*, November, Special Table B, XXIV-XLV. Washington, D.C.: United Nations.

————. 1974a. Paper presented at World Population Conference, Bucharest, Rumania, August 1974. World Population Year Bulletin 16. New York: United Nations Fund for Population Activities.

————. 1974b. Report of the Symposium on Population and Human Rights, Amsterdam. World Population Year Bulletin 16. New York: United Nations Fund for Population Activities.

————. 1980. World Fertility Survey Conference, London, 7 July 1980.

Wagley, C. 1957. Plantation America: a culture sphere. In *Caribbean Studies: A Symposium*, ed. V. Rubin, pp. 3-13. Kingston: Institute of Social and Economic Research, University of the West Indies.

Walsh, B. T. 1970. *Economic development and population control: a fifty-year projection for Jamaica*. London: Praeger.

West India Royal Commission Report. 1945. London: Her Majesty's Stationery Office.

Williamson, J. B. 1970. Subjective efficacy and ideal family size as predictions of favorability toward birth control. *Demography* 7:329-339.

Wolf, E. R. 1959. Specific aspects of plantation systems of the new world: community subcultures and social classes. *Social Science Monograph* 7:136-146. Washington, D.C.: Pan American University.

World Health Assembly. 1979. WHO long-term programme for maternal and child health. Geneva: World Health Organization.

World Health Organization. 1973. *Health education in health aspects of family planning*. Technical Report Series, no. 483. Geneva: World Health Organization.

Zelnick, M., and J. Kanter. First pregnancies in women aged 15-19: 1976 and 1978. *Family Planning Perspectives* 10:11.

Index

Abortifacients, 45-48
Abortion, 50-52
Abstinence, 48-49
Action patterns. See Group action
  patterns
Africa: culture of, 52-55; as socio-
  political symbol, 55-58; and Jamaican culture, 188-192
Age: and contraception, 92-99, 110-
  112, 118; personal meaning of, 99-
  100; of menarche and first coitus,
  124-125, 139, 155; of first union, 151,
  155, 156; of first pregnancy, 153-158
  passim; and conjugal stability, 194-
  195, 204; and marriage status, 253-
  255
Aloe vera, 50
Annona muricata, 44
Attitudes: male-dominant, 116-117,
  147-148; and socioeconomic status,
  117-118; matricentric, 132, 138, 142,
  143, 192-194, 251, 256-257; fertility-
  related, 169-172
Autonomy, personal, 222-225, 235,
  237, 239. See also Self-esteem

Babylon theme, 63-64
Balm yards, 53, 54
Beaubrun, Michael, 23, 24
Bedward, Alexander, 107
Behavior. See Group action patterns;
  Sexual-reproductive behavior
Birth, urban and rural, 98, 101-102
Birth control, 7-8, 24-25; ambivalence

toward, 84-85, 248. See also Contra-
  ceptive use; Family planning; Fertil-
  ity regulation; Population control;
  Population policy; Public policy
Birthrate, 1-2; in Jamaica, 8-9, 24, 68
Black power, 55-58
Blacks: in Baltimore, 5, 23; premarital
  births of, 187; as rural class, 190;
  male, status of, 191
Body, folk approach to, 59-60
Botanical substances, 43-47, 59
British: and Jamaican identity, 56;
  colonial power of, 188-189, 232;
  women, reproductive-contraceptive
  behavior of, 238-239
Bush teas, 40-41, 44, 45, 50, 261

Calabash, 46-47
Categories, shared. See Group action
  patterns
Cerasee, 45, 46
Chemicals, for fertility regulation, 47-
  48, 59
Childbearing. See Children; Parenthood; Pregnancy
Childhood, of female respondents, 132-
  134, 141-145
Child rearing, and reproductive
  behavior, 141-145
Children, 4-5; value of, 4, 91, 118-119,
  152, 164-166, 169-170, 252; vulnerability of, 87-92; malnutrition of, 88,
  240; first, 172-173, 176-185; "passing on" of, 173-176, 182, 183; uncon-

scious resentment of, 182, 183. *See also* Parenthood; Pregnancy

Church attendance, 106-109, 112. *See also* Religion

Class structure. *See* Socioeconomic organization

Client-patients, 79-81. *See also* Respondents, female; Respondents, male

Clinics, 12, 13, 259; East Street, 12, 13, 33, 79; Manley, 18, 34, 79-80

Cohabiting, 190, 195, 198, 204-206

Coitus. *See* Intercourse

Coitus interruptus, 49

Collective action patterns. *See* Group action patterns

Colonialism, 188-189, 232

Communication: couple, 249, 256-258; public policy for, 253-259. *See also* Instruction, sexual-reproductive; Mates, communication with; Mothers, daughters' relationship with

Competence, 209-222 passim. *See also* Autonomy, personal

Condom, use of, 109-117. *See also* Contraceptive use

Conflict, unconscious, in female respondents, 181-185

Conflict resolution: first coitus as, 143, 144, 242; as group action pattern, 242-243

Contraceptive use: psychosocial barriers to, 13-14; interviews on, 33-38; attitudes toward, 42, 43, 59, 84-85, 96-99, 109-118, 248; government attitude toward, 84-85, 141-142, 237; of female respondents, 92-99, 117-118, 155-166, 243-244; early, late, and consistency of, 92-94; male, 109-118, 141, 177-181, 243; and non-use, 160-166, 244; in Pakistan, 236; and autonomy and personal efficacy, 236-237, 239, 242; class differences and, 238-239; in U.S., 248-249; indigenous and acceptable methods of, 248, 260-262. *See also* Birth control; Fertility regulation; Sexual-reproductive behavior

Coping, 222-225

Counseling, 260

Couple communication, 249, 256-258. *See also* Mates, communication and satisfaction with

Culture: interactions in, 15-16; African, 52-58; change and, 95-99, 251-252, 256-259; Afro-Jamaican, 189-192; integrity of, 231-234; Jamaican, and reproductive policy, 250-253. *See also* Africa; Jamaica

Cunnilingus, 50

Data, statistical analysis of, 38

Daughters: relationship with mothers, 129-144, 153-155, 160, 169, 181-185, 193-194, 216, 240-244 passim, 251, 258; value of, 164-166. *See also* Children; Motherhood, culture of

David, Henry, 25

Defense and coping, 222-225

Deprivation, childhood, 133-134

Discipline, 133-138 passim. *See also* Instruction, sexual-reproductive; Mothers, daughters' relationship with

Doctors, 18-20, 26-32

Douches, 48

Draw-a-person performance, 219-222

East Street Clinic. *See* Clinics

Economics, as factor in sexual-reproductive behavior, 82-92, 94, 98, 112-118. *See also* Socioeconomic organization

Education, 10-11; and contraception, 88-90, 96-98, 102-104, 105; of female respondents, 88-90, 96-98, 102-104, 105, 117-118, 138, 212-213; of male respondents, 113-115, 117-118; and modernity, 237-238. *See also* Instruction, sexual-reproductive

Emigration. *See* Migration

Employment, and self-esteem, 4, 90, 234-235. *See also* Occupation; Unemployment

Ethel A., 62-64

Ethnographer. *See* Participant-observer

Family context: of female respondents, 129-138, 141-145, 169-170; of male respondents, 138-141; and unconscious conflict, 181-185

Family of origin: and induced cultural change, 256-259; and counseling, 260

Family planning, 7-14 passim, 232-233, 237, 239, 247-253; ambivalence toward, 84-85; in Pakistan, 236; services and workers, 259-262

Family stability: public policy for, 253-259; counseling for, 260

Family structure, historical roots of, 188-192

Fathers: adolescent, 6; female respondents' relationship with, 130-132

Favelas, 4, 22

Fellatio, 50

Female respondents. See Respondents, female

Fertility, 2, 49-61, 68; government policy on, 7-8, 232-233, 237, 239, 247-253; African influences on, 52-55, 57-58; shared categories and private meanings of, 58-61; attitudes related to, 169-172. See also Sexual-reproductive behavior

Fertility regulation: personal, 8, 25, 41-43, 48-49, 248; technological, 16-17; nondrug, 42-43; botanical substances and chemicals for, 47-48, 59; natural, 58-59, 260-261. See also Birth control; Contraceptive use; Family planning; Population control; Population policy; Public policy

Flogging, 133-134, 135-136

Folk categories and meanings, 58-61

Folk culture, African influences on, 52-55. See also Africa; Culture; Jamaica

Garvey, Marcus, 55, 57

Government fertility policy. See Population policy; Public policy

Grandmothers, role of, 129, 130, 132, 138, 140, 141, 170, 183, 206, 213-214, 244, 251. See also Attitudes, matricentric

Group action patterns, 16, 31, 242-243; and private meanings, 58-61; symptomatic, 225-230, 242-243, 244; and conflict resolution, 242-243

Guiacum officinale, 41

Healers, folk, 53-55

Health policy, public, 247, 249-250

Household arrangements, 199-200. See also Unions, conjugal

Housing, 78-81, 88. See also Residence patterns

Immigration. See Migration

Infants: mortality rate, 84; malnutrition of, 88, 240. See also Children

Informants, cultural map of, 15. See also Client-patients; Respondents, female; Respondents, male

Instruction, sexual-reproductive, 133-138 passim, 141, 142, 155-164 passim, 241-242, 244, 249, 258

Intercourse: anal, 49; attitudes toward, 59; male frequency of, 110, 112; first, 124-144 passim, 150-152, 155, 156, 184, 242, 243-244; symptomatic, 225-230, 242. See also Sexual-reproductive behavior

Interviewer. See Participant-observer

Interviewing, 31-38

Investigator. See Participant-observer

Jamaica, 22, 23, 64-68; socioeconomic organization of, 20-21, 189-190, 231-234, 238; population distribution in, 67-68. See also Culture

Jamaica Family Planning Association (JFPA), 12, 259

Jamaica Family Planning League, 12

Kingston, 63-64, 69, 70, 72-75; residence patterns in, 75-79; housing conditions in, 78-81, 88

Knowledge, reproductive, 160-164. See also Education; Instruction, sexual-reproductive; Literacy

Kumina, 52-53

Lactation: prolonged, 41, 42, 48; and

infant malnutrition, 240
Land and land tenure, 66-67, 190
Lewin, Olive, 40, 41, 52, 53, 106
Lignum vitae, 40, 41
Literacy: campaign, 88-90; of female respondents, 212-213. See also Education

Magico-religious acts, 60
Males: dominant attitudes, 116-117, 147-148; black, status of, 191; attitudes toward, 192-194, 195, 244. See also Mates; Respondents, male
Malnutrition, 2; infant, 88, 240
Marigold, symbolism of, 30, 45
Marijuana, 41, 66
Marriage: and pregnancy, 186-188, 254-255; attitudes toward, 192-194, 195, 244; and age, 253-255. See also Unions, conjugal
Mates: communication and satisfaction with, 129, 132, 133, 151, 155-160 passim, 169, 188, 195-196, 233, 242, 244, 249, 256-258 passim; first, 150-152, 154-160, 244
Medical centers, 10-11. See also Clinics; Doctors; Patients
Medicine, folk, 40-41, 43-47
Menarche, 30, 45, 46; feelings about, 59, 124-131 passim, 240-242
Migration: global, 2; circular, 2, 95; in Jamaica, 69-70; external, 100-101, 142; internal, 101, 190
Modernization, 234-240, 262
Montego Bay, 68, 78-79
Motherhood, culture of, 237, 244, 251, 256-257. See also Attitudes, matricentric; Mothers, daughters' relationship with
Mothers: adolescent, 5; vulnerability of, 87-92; daughters' relationship with, 129-132, 136-138, 142-144 passim, 153-155 passim, 160, 169, 181-185, 193-194, 216, 240-242, 244, 251, 258; sons' relationship with, 140, 141, 258
Mulatto class, 189

Nanas, 45, 46, 259

National Family Planning Board (NFPB), 12
Nationalism, in Jamaica, 231-234
Neighborhoods. See Housing; Residence patterns; Shantytowns
Nettleford, Rex M., 24, 63
Nutrition. See Health policy, public; Lactation; Malnutrition

Obeah, 29, 30, 32, 49, 54
Occupation, 90-92; and contraceptive use, 90-91, 99-100, 104-106; aspirations, 216. See also Employment; Unemployment
Origins and pawns, 236-237

Parenthood, 5-7, 87-88, 141-145; and self-esteem, 4, 87, 91, 119. See also Sexual-reproductive behavior
Participant-observer: comprehension of, 15, 17, 26; social role of, 17-21; as physician, 18, 19-20, 26-31; person of, 21-26
Partner diversity, 200-208
Partnership, sexual. See Mates; Unions, conjugal
"Passing on," 173-176, 182, 183
Patients, 26, 79-81; relationship with doctor, 19-20, 26-31, 32
Patterns, group. See Group action patterns
Pennyroyal, 45-46
Plantation societies, 231-234
Population: African, 52; Jamaican, 67-68; in Kingston, 69, 72
Population control, global, 24-25
Population growth, 1-4
Population policy, 7-8, 232-233, 237, 239, 247-253. See also Contraceptive use; Public policy
Potency, 49-61
Poverty, 4-5, 23. See also Socioeconomic organization
Pregnancy, 92-95, 137-139, 144-150, 184, 244-246; first, 151-160, 166-172, 181, 184, 185, 244; attitudes toward, 166-172; reconstitutive function of, 181-182; and marriage, 186-188, 254-155; and partner diversity, 200,

206; and maternal relationship, 241

Private meanings, and shared categories, 58-61. *See also* Group action patterns

Public policy, 247-250, 262; reproductive, 250-253, 258; for family stability and communication, 257-259. *See also* Contraceptive use; Population policy

Public symbols, and private meanings, 60-61. *See also* Group action patterns

Purges, 47-48

Race. *See* Culture; Socioeconomic organization

Ram-goat dashalong, 47

Rastafarians, 55-58, 63, 76-77

Refugees, 3. *See also* Migration

Reggae, 84, 86

Religion, 60, 106-109, 232

Reproduction: global crisis of, 1-8; universal right of, 7-8, 248; folk ideas about, 58-61. *See also* Sexual-reproductive behavior

Residence patterns, 75-78. *See also* Housing

Respondents, female, 92-109, 124-125; socioeconomic status of, 83-92, 94, 98, 139; contraceptive status of, 92-95, 137-139 passim, 144-145, 244; affective flatness of, 209-222 passim; self-presentation of, 211-212; mood of, 213-216. *See also* Contraceptive use; Daughters; Menarche; Mothers; Sexual-reproductive behavior

Respondents, male, 109-118, 138-141, 176-181, 204-208, 243

Revivalism, 107

Ritual baths, 53

Rural birth, 98, 101-102

Rural-urban differences, 189-190

St. Andrew Parish, 70-72

Sampling, 31-38

Schools, 88-90. *See also* Education

Self-concept, modern, 234-240, 246

Self-esteem: and employment, 4, 90,

234-235; and sexual-reproductive behavior, 4, 87, 91, 119, 130, 234-239 passim. *See also* Autonomy, personal

Sempervivum, 50

Sex, folk ideas about, 58-61

Sex education. *See* Contraceptive use; Family planning; Instruction, sexual-reproductive; Knowledge, reproductive

Sexual-reproductive behavior, 17, 92-100, 109-118; symptomatic, 225-230, 242-243; social context of, 231-240; scenario, 243-247. *See also* Contraceptive use; Group action patterns; Intercourse; Pregnancy; Respondents, female; Respondents, male

Shantytowns, 78-79

Shepherds, balm yard, 53, 54

Sinkle-Bible, 50

Slavery, 188-191

Slums. *See* Housing; Residence patterns

Socioeconomic organization, 20-21, 189-190, 231-234, 238; and class dissonance, 22, 34, 73; and sexual-reproductive behavior, 82-92, 94, 98-100, 112-118, 139, 238-239

Soursop, 44

Spanish Town, 68

Spirit healing, 53

Statistics, gamma, 38

Stillbirths, 51

Subjects, 15. *See also* Respondents, female; Respondents, male

Symbols, public, and private meanings, 60-61. *See also* Group action patterns, symptomatic

Teas, 40-41, 44, 45, 50, 261

Thematic Apperception Test cards, 216-219

Thyme, 47

Towns and country, differences between, 189-190

Traditions, African, 52-55. *See also* Africa; Culture

Turnera ulmifolia, 47

Unemployment, 90-92, 104-106; and
  population growth, 3-4; in Baltimore, 5. *See also* Employment;
  Occupation
Unions, conjugal, 10, 194-199, 253-256;
  first, 150-152, 154-160, 186, 245;
  visiting, 190, 195, 196-197, 204-205,
  243, 253-255; cohabiting, 198, 204-
  206, 253-255; duration of, 198-199;
  of male respondents, 204-206. *See
  also* Couple communication; Marriage; Mates

Urban birth, 98, 101-102
Urban-rural differences, 189-190

Values, 10-11
Visiting, 190, 195, 196-197, 204-205,
  243

Washouts, 45, 47, 48
World Health Organization (WHO),
  7-8, 23